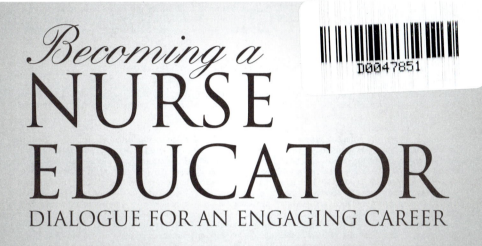

Becoming a NURSE EDUCATOR

DIALOGUE FOR AN ENGAGING CAREER

CeCelia R. Zorn, PhD, RN

Professor
College of Nursing and Health Sciences
University of Wisconsin–Eau Claire
Eau Claire, Wisconsin

JONES AND BARTLETT PUBLISHERS

Sudbury, Massachusetts

BOSTON   TORONTO   LONDON   SINGAPORE

World Headquarters

Jones and Bartlett Publishers
40 Tall Pine Drive
Sudbury, MA 01776
978-443-5000
info@jbpub.com
www.jbpub.com

Jones and Bartlett Publishers
Canada
6339 Ormindale Way
Mississauga, Ontario L5V 1J2
Canada

Jones and Bartlett Publishers
International
Barb House, Barb Mews
London W6 7PA
United Kingdom

Jones and Bartlett's books and products are available through most bookstores and online booksellers. To contact Jones and Bartlett Publishers directly, call 800-832-0034, fax 978-443-8000, or visit our website, www.jbpub.com.

Substantial discounts on bulk quantities of Jones and Bartlett's publications are available to corporations, professional associations, and other qualified organizations. For details and specific discount information, contact the special sales department at Jones and Bartlett via the above contact information or send an email to specialsales@jbpub.com.

The author, editor, and publisher have made every effort to provide accurate information. However, they are not responsible for errors, omissions, or for any outcomes related to the use of the contents of this book and take no responsibility for the use of the products and procedures described. Treatments and side effects described in this book may not be applicable to all people; likewise, some people may require a dose or experience a side effect that is not described herein. Drugs and medical devices are discussed that may have limited availability controlled by the Food and Drug Administration (FDA) for use only in a research study or clinical trial. Research, clinical practice, and government regulations often change the accepted standard in this field. When consideration is being given to use of any drug in the clinical setting, the health care provider or reader is responsible for determining FDA status of the drug, reading the package insert, and reviewing prescribing information for the most up-to-date recommendations on dose, precautions, and contraindications, and determining the appropriate usage for the product. This is especially important in the case of drugs that are new or seldom used.

Production Credits
Publisher: Kevin Sullivan
Acquisitions Editor: Emily Ekle
Acquisitions Editor: Amy Sibley
Associate Editor: Patricia Donnelly
Editorial Assistant: Rachel Shuster
Senior Production Editor: Carolyn F. Rogers
Senior Marketing Manager: Barb Bartoszek
V.P., Manufacturing and Inventory Control: Therese Connell
Composition: Toppan Best-set Typesetter Ltd., Hong Kong
Cover Design: Kristin E. Parker
Cover Image: © Sarkao/Dreamstime.com
Printing and Binding: Malloy, Inc.
Cover Printing: Malloy, Inc.

Library of Congress Cataloging-in-Publication Data
Zorn, CeCelia R.
    Becoming a nurse educator : dialogue for an engaging career / CeCelia R. Zorn.
        p. ; cm.
    Includes bibliographical references and index.
    ISBN 978-0-7637-7111-9 (pbk.)
1. Nursing—Study and teaching.   I. Title.
    [DNLM: 1. Education, Nursing.   2. Teaching—methods.   WY 18 Z88b 2010]
    RT71.Z67 2010
    610.73—dc22
                                    2009016100

6048

Printed in the United States of America
13 12 11 10 09   10 9 8 7 6 5 4 3 2 1

Dedication

To all the students who have been my teachers—you have walked by my side with style and goodwill. You helped me hear the songs of a different flute.

Contents

Foreword

When I was a much younger man, I became a nurse. The moment of decision was impulsive and incidental (what decision made by a 17-year-old is not?), but then again I had been studying the humane arts at the foot of my mother since the day I first began forming memories. A registered nurse by training, certification, and calling, my mother left the hospital early, folding her profession into our everyday life by taking in all manner of sick and sometimes dying children. My siblings and I came of age in a farmhouse medical ward, and as the eldest son, over the course of my first 17 years I was often dubbed mother's lieutenant on trips to the more formal halls of medicine. I grew up with the sound of the oxygen tank bubbling, came of age holding tiny hands in the recovery room, learned early the language of medicine and malady. In many practical respects, this informal apprenticeship gave me a head start on nursing school. I had seen the stitches. Changed the dressings. Helped draw the dose.

And yet I was unaware of what it meant to *become* a nurse. My mother knew, of course, but it took the benevolent (and let us not soft-pedal it: *rigorous*) intervention of my nursing instructors over the course of 4 years to penetrate the blithe inattention of my youth, to help me understand that to *become* a nurse I would need to raise my eyes from the sphygmomanometer and the vitals chart and consider horizons far beyond the medicine cart.

Ours was a nursing program based on a paradigm of holistic patient care. I clearly recall chafing at what I perceived as the wifty-wafty aspects of this concept, just as I chafed at the humanity electives I was required to take. I considered them a superfluous indulgence of time better spent learning to thread a feeding tube or assess skin turgor. And yet, staying their course, my instructors punctured my preconceptions one pinhole at a time, each time letting in new light that struck me from angles I had not previously considered. For instance, it one day dawned on me that far from residing wholly in the ineffable theoretical, holistic assessment—by its very definition—also got down and wallowed in the grittiest of the nitty-gritty.

Perhaps the term *punctured* as used above is inapt. The greatest power of an instructor is not to inject learning, but rather to draw the learner out. While reading the text of the book you are holding, I was struck time and time again by how completely I had failed to previously consider the part preparation, dedication, and hope played in the composition of the lectures I absorbed all those years ago. For the best of my professors, the syllabus was simply the framework upon which to construct a much more ornate—one could say *holistic*—tapestry. When I emerged from the program, my perception of nursing had been expanded and transformed to a degree that would alter my perceptions of life itself. This is not an overstatement. In fact, in what may or may not be an endorsement for this book, those very same instructors set me on a path in which I wound up supporting myself largely outside the medical world. Their dedication to the spirituality of learning, to the integration of many parts into the whole, put me on a journey that for all its meandering is strung from threads that can be traced directly back to nursing instructors who cared enough to compel me to consider nursing beyond the toes of my white shoes. By the same token, it is their lasting influence that has kept me involved—even if on a volunteer basis—in health care for the past 20 years even as my avocations took me outside the professional realm.

The foundation of nursing must rest forever on solid skills. This is primary, and paramount. My instructors saw to this, and to this day, if need be, I can catheterize you in a trice. But if this book is to serve its purpose, it will inspire student and teacher alike to strive for an education that cultivates nurses with the potential to supplement physical intervention with an engaged humanity toward all humanity. Having witnessed that spirit in the nursing instructors who still shape me, I remain, even now, even after all the twists and turns that followed my time in their classrooms, privileged and grateful to sign my name.

Michael Perry, RN

Introduction

As an emerging nurse educator you have been admitted to a graduate program and are eagerly pursuing a long-held aspiration.

Or as a new nursing faculty you have already assembled a hefty collection of nursing education books, pored over multiple teaching/learning theories in recent graduate classes, and fretfully practiced some "creative" teaching strategies.

Or you just signed a contract to teach during the next semester but never had an education course or opened an education book (and your stunned nurse practitioner friends raise a wary eyebrow, "You did *what*?").

Or you have recently completed a Doctorate in Nursing Practice program where you have been submerged in practice and systems coursework and now are beginning a first-time teaching position with minimal exposure to education as a discipline.

Or you are finishing doctoral dissertation research, triumphant but exhausted and now primed to further cultivate your role as an educator.

Or you've just finished teaching your first jarring semester as an instructional academic staff and, feeling a bit fragile, tentatively read the student evaluations.

Or you are a time-honored faculty, long-established but searching for meaning in your own teaching and learning as you contemplate how you and your ideas may attend colleagues new to nursing education.

Becoming a Nurse Educator: Dialogue for an Engaging Career is here to serve you. This book sifts through the human side of teaching, its daily-ness. It will enrich your venture into nursing education or offer a reflection on your seasoned career. The principal goal is to help new faculty embrace nursing education as liberal education, shifting away from a "professional studies" emphasis that simply adds to a compilation of disparate general education courses. Nursing education as liberal education accomplishes more than merely preparing a nurse or emphasizing workforce development—liberal nursing education prepares a person and teaches life. This shift is essential before constructive changes can occur in our current healthcare system and around the world.

ASSUMPTIONS AND ASPIRATIONS

This book is based on the assumption that teaching is a unique discipline. Teaching does not necessarily come naturally; that is, just because one is an expert clinician or administrator or researcher or student does not mean that one instinctively is a skilled teacher. To help new nursing faculty craft nursing education more fully as liberal education, I concentrate on three explicit purposes: (1) affirm educators in their transition to the faculty role, (2) uncover meaning in becoming an educator, and (3) examine relationships with students and teaching practices that redesign nursing education as liberal education. Realizing this goal demands a public discourse about teaching—it mandates that we unwrap a dialogue in a way that has not been our habit or our history.

Bringing teaching openly into the commons for exchange and conversation, particularly for the new educator, inspired me to write this book built on the town commons as metaphor. The commons is an area where individuals and groups both draw from and add to.

There is a centrality and sincerity to the commons, a resource available to all that both generates and extends our work. The commons is cooperatively built and maintained; it is the impetus for both big breakthroughs as well as the less glamorous incremental innovations. The commons makes public that which is often extremely private. With this book, I hope to open doors rather than to close them.

To center teaching in our town commons, I have interwoven my stories, experiences, and reflections from 30 years in nursing education with the popular and professional literature to create the structure for the book. Using a personal, narrative, experiential approach (dashed with jest, spiked with self-deprecation, and edged with a bit of sting), I urge new faculty to identify and shape what are meaning and style for them.

This soul side of teaching within an expansive liberal education is fundamental for the beginning nurse educator and yet this is what is missing in the existing literature. I could find no other book that is specifically directed to new faculty. Although other books claim a general application to both the novice and seasoned educator, little text in those books speaks directly, thoroughly, and earnestly to new teachers.

Becoming a Nurse Educator is written primarily for the nurse faculty beginning a position in an academic setting or in transition to that role. This individual may be currently enrolled in graduate education courses or have recently completed a master's or doctoral degree and now is launching an academic teaching position. Or the new faculty may be a seasoned graduate degree–prepared nurse with a lengthy and specialized practice history and now is changing career roles and moving into higher education for the first time. Last, there is also a growing number of part-time nurse educators new to the academic setting. They often hold concurrent practice positions and have had little formal preparation for the educator role.

As novice faculty, all of these nurses come to teaching with lofty educational accomplishments and well-developed clinical expertise. But they frequently come with little or no experience as nurse educators and, more often than not, receive minimal preceptorship or mentorship in their teaching position.

Becoming a Nurse Educator helps fulfill a critical need as we see growing numbers of new nursing faculty, with the trend expected to continue. Early retirements, economically driven exits from academe, and an aging faculty retiring within the next decade contribute to increasing faculty vacancy rates.

At the same time there is also an increase in the need for faculty. Because of the existing nursing shortage and the likelihood that it will continue, many legislators, alumni, and university fund-raising leaders are paying more attention and providing more financial support to nursing education than ever before. Not only are the traditional education programs often admitting more students, but also more nontraditional options are being created (e.g., accelerated programs for second-degree students, fast-tracking programs for a baccalaureate-to-doctorate degree, and expanding doctorate in nursing practice programs). All of these expansions call for more nursing faculty.

Hence, on the one hand, faculty vacancy rates are increasing because of faculty exits and retirements. On the other hand, demands for faculty are increasing simultaneously as many nursing education programs are expanding in response to the national nursing shortage. As a result of existing and projected nursing faculty shortages, then, nursing programs, university administrators, and faculty are increasingly emphasizing the preparation, recruitment, and retention of new nurse educators.

Increasing faculty preparation, recruitment, and retention are not restricted to activities in the United States alone; there is also a concentrated focus to establish and expand nursing education around the world. In several areas internationally, this expansion is also changing from a technical, workforce development approach to nursing preparation that is university-based and more liberal in focus.

Becoming a Nurse Educator can be used singly or in combination with other texts in various ways. For example, the book could serve as (1) a course text in master's or doctoral classes in nursing or other disciplines (e.g., educational leadership) where nurses are examining or preparing for the faculty role in an academic setting, (2) a resource for newly employed full- or part-time nursing faculty (and their supervisors and personnel committee members), in faculty development workshops, or within formal or informal preceptor programs or mentoring relationships, and (3) a guide to introduce the educator role to nurses in practice who are contemplating pursuing a graduate degree or students already enrolled in graduate programs as they deliberate role preparation.

In addition to use by new and emerging educators in the United States and internationally, experienced teachers may also use *Becoming a Nurse Educator* to facilitate their own self-reflection, examining where they have been and how they might move forward. Through this self-reflection, perhaps they can counsel others joining our ranks in ways that are worthwhile for the new educator, enriching for themselves, and beneficial for the profession and health care more broadly.

The book can be used in its entirety or by reading selected units or chapters, here and there, at the end of a demanding day or a wearing week. Both individuals and groups who meet in face-to-face or online discussions will find that the writings enlarge and clarify experiences or evoke and affirm feelings.

To be clear, *Becoming a Nurse Educator* is not a handbook, or an instructor's manual prescribing rigid and canned "how-to-teach" strategies that all educators must use to be successful. Neither is the goal to present a complete literature review of education research and theory or describe curriculum development and evaluation.

BOOK OVERVIEW

Four units have been designed to summon the novice faculty to our teaching commons. First, "Knowing the Self as Teacher" invites the new faculty to pause and reflect: *Who am I that teaches? Where have I been? What is important to me? How am I continuing my life as a learner and beginning my life as a teacher?* In the second unit, "Relationships With Students," the students' voice leads teaching and learning. Following the distinction given to students, several teaching approaches with detailed examples are offered in the third unit, "Teaching Practices That I Am Practicing." Rooted in my experiences, these approaches are often fledgling, forever emerging. The final unit, "Nursing Education as Liberal Education" moves us beyond merely "teaching the work" of nursing and draws us closer to "teaching life" with nurses.

Teaching *what* to think propels the former whereas teaching *how* to think draws the latter.

Unit 1, "Knowing the Self as Teacher," has five chapters. In Chapter 1, "Then and Now: A Call to Pause," I briefly review my own educational journey and career trajectory, and examine the need to pause and reflect. Pausing in self-reflection is particularly critical for new faculty transitioning to academe. Both the benefits of pause and its challenges in our culture are discussed. They are grounded in the writings of Alice Walker, Amy Tan, and Carol Shields, as well as in my personal experience with an English-Swedish translation and the use of a Key West sunset as metaphor for crossing a threshold. References to poetry and art, an Einstein quote, and ideas from Parker Palmer are used to find who we are and describe the delicate process of going inside that is required. Cherry Ames, the 1960s fictional book series about nursing, is used to introduce and conclude the chapter, providing the then and now orientation.

The focus of the second chapter in Unit 1, "Honoring the Present in the Best and Worst Year," is cherishing how we learn and develop as teachers and the need to "forgive and remember." The chapter's foundation is a first-year nurse educator's essay written in a graduate course in which she describes being told by her hiring supervisor that the first year would be "icky," to be expected, and things would get better. New faculty will see themselves in this essay summary, as well as in the research describing first-year teaching experiences and Lee Shulman's comparison of new to experienced teachers. Several metaphors are used to illustrate the paradox of being planted in the mud and muck of daily existence as a new teacher and a new employee and yet, at the same time, feeling restless, stretching and growing. My own evolution as an educator is described in considerable detail, using Palmer's and Annie Dillard's ideas about knowing the self and internalizing a role.

The third chapter in this unit continues to use the first year of teaching as a springboard for launching an engaging career in nursing education. "'As If': More of That First Year" presumes that a smoldering, internal confidence anchors who we are as new teachers. To sustain this "as if" centeredness, the perspectives of two new nurse educators and my own reflections are used to explore issues that consistently surface for novice faculty: (1) appeal of the educator role, (2) preparing to teach, (3) getting started, and (4) relationships with teaching colleagues. This discussion builds on the previous chapter where wide-ranging abstract metaphors illustrate the first year; here, many specific techniques and approaches are offered.

"Scott's Spirit on Lassen Peak: Finding the Spirit That Sustains You" is the fourth chapter in the unit. Instead of the dull and frequently impossible way to find balance in life, the thesis in this chapter is that a critical venture for the new faculty is to discover what it is that sustains you—what is the spirit that motivates you and is your source of power? Modified from Whyte's writing, the difference between spirit and strategy is described. Learning about spirit from Scott, a 3-year-old climbing Lassen Peak, provides the basis for the discussion. The majority of the chapter is about learning; learning is framed as the spirit for me—learning sustains me. I describe five dimensions that I've learned about learning as they emerge from my own experiences: (1) learning delights and stimulates, (2) learning heightens confidence, (3) learning "lightens up," (4) learning helps us see the flipside, and (5) learning wakes up a bonus or a premium. My intent is that not only will new faculty begin to examine spirit for themselves (i.e., what sustains them), but also expand their own conceptualization of learning and then, of course, how students regard learning.

The final chapter in Unit 1 is "The Rhythm of Education: Dr. Harriet Werley, Thank You for Teaching Me." The goal in this chapter is to use my experiences to explore mentorship and how it can form teaching throughout one's life. Dr. Harriet Werley's mentorship when I was a doctoral student was threefold, and I describe it as Rhythms of Education: (1) Rhythm of Staccato (teaching me to be rigorous, teach with definition, define a central story), (2) Rhythm of Tapestry (teaching me to relate, connect, teach with synthesis and integration), and (3) Rhythm of Stillness (teaching me to be affirming, life-giving, valuing silence and solitude).

Unit 2, "Relationships With Students," has two chapters. In the first, "How Can the Students Help Us Teach?" the students' voice leads a discussion about teaching. Remarks from an informal interview with two students center on the following areas: (1) characteristics of nursing students, (2) teacher characteristics that are helpful and less helpful, and (3) suggestions for new faculty. I've used the students' perspective to integrate my own teaching and learning experiences in this chapter.

"Presence With Students: Posing Interest, Not Merely Paying Attention" is the second chapter in Unit 2. Joyce Carol Oates described Alice James as a career-invalid with a myriad of physical and emotional ailments. James's family heaped piles of *attention* on her, but she was the focus of no one's *interest*. This description is used to discuss the idea that establishing presence with students is not merely paying attention—it is posing interest. First, a clinical teaching experience when I was a new faculty is used to show how students taught me the difference between paying attention and posing interest. This was a watershed in my understanding of teaching and student–teacher relationships; how my approach to relationships changed is described. A second example from my preceptorship with a teaching colleague is used to discuss posing interest in the classroom. Examples of posing interest from Abraham Lincoln's presidency are highlighted and linked to what we do as teachers. Specific strategies in providing feedback, as a key component in posing interest, are offered.

Four chapters comprise Unit 3: "Teaching Practices That I Am Practicing." After each chapter in this unit, I have used some Socratic techniques to pose several discussion questions. These "questions to ponder" ask for clarification, probe assumptions, call for evidence, invite other perspectives, examine consequences, and study the question itself.

The first chapter, "Clinical Teaching Is Where the Magic Lies," uses Jeffrey Kluger's Complexity Arc to describe the delicate balance that characterizes clinical teaching—the balance between panic and gridlock. In this chapter, several strategies are highlighted that emphasize the significance of preparation, as well as specific guidelines to consider throughout the semester. For example, establishing and maintaining relationships with colleagues and students, helping students learn to think, and prioritizing key concepts are illustrated.

The second chapter in this unit is "The Novel: 'Listen Her and She Will Show Us Everything'." Reading a novel can unsettle uncertainties students often have about others. It shakes us up and makes us question our truths. Responses of human beings, as the core of nursing, are linked with novel reading. This chapter uses Pamela Gien's *The Syringa Tree* and Carol Shield's *Unless* as examples to show that novel reading can help us strip away the surface and explain what is underneath and also appreciate how people connect with each other. Benefits of novel reading in a liberal nursing education are discussed (e.g., granting voice, discovering systems, understanding prevention). Explicitly geared toward novice faculty, substantial "how-to's" of using novel reading in teaching are also described. An example of a student's thinking and writing around Jeffrey Eugenides's *Middlesex* illustrates a class assignment. An anecdote from Lincoln's childhood, as told by Richard Slotkin in his historical novel, poignantly concludes the chapter and begs us to "listen her and she will show us everything."

Continuing the discussion about teaching practices, the third chapter in Unit 3 is "Students Co-Construct the Classroom." Students' discussion creates a vivid classroom experience for both the learner and the teacher. Inviting and incorporating students' comments in the classroom are particularly difficult for the new faculty, as often the novice teacher is tethered to her or his lecture notes, nearly having a planned script for the class presentation. In addition, the new faculty is frequently teaching content that is less familiar and may be painfully uncomfortable with silence. One detailed classroom example where students' discussion was encouraged is used to illustrate teaching approaches that tend to be much more effective, compared to the same classroom example where teacher approaches worked less well. In this example comparison, "accountable talk," use of students' names, ways that pauses can be used successfully, and useful strategies in preparing for class are described in detail

"Creative Projects: 'Could You Please Tell Us What You're Looking For?'" is the final chapter in the unit. Admirably, most novice teachers are highly motivated to "be creative," seeing this as one of the pleasurable aspects of their teaching. For many, however, the technique is daunting, their skills are minimal, and they receive little support from their colleagues (being told that "creativity is frosting on the cake"). The goal of this chapter is to help new faculty incorporate creative projects in their teaching. My own early experiences in using creative projects and why they did not really work are presented. Following a brief theoretical description of creativity in education a more effective classroom example is provided. In this detailed before-and-after description of a creative project in teaching leadership content, several teaching techniques are examined: (1) introducing creativity to the students, (2) helping students see themselves in the phases of creativity development, (3) highlighting Sign and Design and helping students use both effectively, and (4) linking the creative project with writing and class discussion.

Unit 4, "Nursing Education as Liberal Education," concludes the book. W. E. B. DuBois's quote about "preparing a man, not a psychologist or a brickmason," as well as his appeal for educators to "teach life, not work" serve as the context for the book's final chapter. Nursing education must *be* a liberal education—teaching life, not education that is added on to a liberal education. Nurse educators must begin to make that mingling and integration. We cannot expect students alone to create that integration, and we cannot expect graduates from nursing programs to be liberally educated if only half their college coursework is indicated or considered as liberal education. Little has been written from that broad perspective; it is my hope that this book will invite more questions and further that dialogue.

Three major sections organize this chapter: (1) beyond compliance in health care, (2) shadow side of present-day nursing education, and (3) nursing education as liberal education. In the first section, Barbara Ehrenreich's *Bait and Switch* is used to discuss an inward-looking, personality-focused, intelligence-minimizing corporate culture. To the extent this culture permeates our healthcare system, the call for a liberally educated nurse—one who is prepared for life, not merely prepared for "work"—is intensified. A heartrending personal example of compliance within health care scaffolds this call.

Several concerns in current nursing education are described in the second section: (1) nursing coursework, as it merely "builds on" general education, and then assumes that a liberally educated nurse is the graduate, and (2) the increasingly popular "cobbling together" of a degree (from multiple college transfers, advanced placement courses in high school, etc.). David Whyte's assertion is connected to this discussion; that is, education is teaching students to conform and preparing employees not to think for themselves.

The final section in this chapter proposes that nursing education as liberal education includes art, agency, and growth. A dialogue with the ideas of Drs. Lee Shulman, Maxine Greene, and John Dewey is used to begin the discussion. Specific examples of teaching strategies are offered to illustrate the three concepts.

The afterword concludes the book. In this closure, I propose that the musicality of teaching demands a lifetime of looking forward and building bridges.

GRACE NOTES AS METAPHOR

As a metaphor, grace notes illustrate the book's foundation. Grace notes are the ornaments of music—they decorate the principal notes and augment the beauty and vigor of the work.

In the same way, *Becoming a Nurse Educator* elaborates what already exists for the beginning faculty; that is, it enlarges the principal notes. First, the novice teacher comes to higher education with expert clinical practice skills and an extensive knowledge of nursing. As a second principal note, the novice teacher also comes as a unique individual with an inherent personal style. Finally, existing literature amply details classroom and clinical teaching and evaluation techniques, content-specific teaching strategies, and curriculum development approaches for nurse faculty.

As a grace note, then, this book builds on the new educators' clinical proficiency and distinctive personhood, and it complements nursing education literature that is already available. It affirms the novice teacher—a "walking with" that embraces both the process of education and the intricate, edgy position of being an educator. A first-person conversational dialogue style serves this affirmation.

In hearing the style and purpose of the book, a colleague indicated that this book could be a "novel among textbooks." As I teach graduate courses in nursing education with students preparing for faculty roles, the types of discussions that are in this book have consistently animated the class. The students have begged me to publish these conversations, describing them as "real . . . showing the fun side of teaching, as well as the challenges . . . it's like you're our coach and we know we'll be successful." One student said, "You don't just tell us a hundred and one strategies to help us 'get the job done,' but you lead us to explore who we are as people, how we are as learners, our lives as educators, how we are becoming a teacher . . . and at the end of the day, we still learn 'how to get the job done.'"

A recent graduate student told me laughingly that the content and style of this book are unique to anything else she had been reading in the nursing education courses. It reminded her of the exercises in her grade school classroom where she was told to "circle the item that does not belong" when presented with several pictures. All of the pictures were related except one. For example, there were all fruits and one vegetable or all tools and one piece of furniture. She needed to circle the vegetable or the piece of furniture to answer the question correctly.

Her observation thrilled us, our talk escalated, and we concluded that people and ideas "that don't belong" are essential. Of course, we instantly realized pain, disadvantage, and marginalization as frequent consequences of power, privilege, and not belonging. However, this book is written in the spirit of being unique, "not belonging," of grace notes that adorn principal notes and turn technique into splendor.

There is a caveat that I must tell you. Considering myself as educator in a formally designated sense feels pretentious and hollow. The very question, *Who am I that teaches?* is a riddle, unanswerable, one that I shrink from. I feel distinctly honored to dare behind my tapestry, as it were, to see my threads in shabby knots and their frayed ends dangling in droops. Thank you for allowing me the privilege of doing that dare with you. Discovering and then speaking about my work have not been easy, but be assured that I have tried my ultimate to be helpful.

So, at the end of the day, when you've just signed your first teaching contract, graded the last essay exam of your first semester teaching, completed the demands of tenure rigor, or taken a moment to reflect on your teaching life, sit back with a steaming cup of ginger tea and read a grace note from *Becoming a Nurse Educator.* You will hear both the harmony and the challenging offbeats of higher education. My hope is that the book is a voice to which you can connect and that it will accent your thoughts, your worries, and your dreams.

Acknowledgments

I am thankful to all who believed I had something to say. And when I doubted myself most, you also helped me see that I had the ability to say it— Mary Ellen Stolder, Marge Bottoms, Sandy Christian, Joanie Stehle Werner, LeeAnna Rasar, Sherri Hydo, Margret Lepp, Karen Solheim, Margaret Gilkison, Maureen Mack, Marcia Bollinger, Bob Lieske, and Chris Weimholt. From the beginning, you stirred ideas in me and unraveled my wonders and my madness with your wisdom.

My gratitude to all the student and teacher voices in this book, but especially Krystle Pagac, Lieneke Hafeman, Diane Marcyjanik, Angie Stombaugh, Kate Lang, Namji Kim, Harriet Werley, and Melissa Anibas. I have seen both your resolve and your flair about teaching and learning. My hope is that I have been true to your word and I beg your pardon for any mis-speak.

And there have been teachers from my grade school and high school that inspired me and kindled my education for life—Mrs. Burgermeister, Mr. Sobeck, Mr. Vogel, Mr. McIlwee, Mr. Bloch, and Mr. and Mrs. Stephenson. They probably wouldn't remember me (and probably tried hard to forget), but I remember them with warm thanks and admiration, and I apologize for my classroom tomfoolery and occasional rowdiness.

My tribute to all nurses—they live the challenges of nursing and health care and yet give everything possible to patients and their colleagues. As liberally educated individuals, they will transform what is yet to come. And I have the valued privilege to be a lifelong student of theirs.

Thank you to the University of Wisconsin–Eau Claire for supporting my sabbatical on two different occasions. I had the treasured opportunity to think, talk, read, write, and play about education. And those sabbaticals would not have been possible without my teaching colleagues who took on ever more each day, each week, while I was away. Please know how grateful I am.

In his book *On Writing*, Stephen King (2000) describes how he opens the door to a piece of his new writing first to a few close friends for their reading and feedback. "You can't let the whole world into your story, but you can let in the ones that matter the most. And you should . . . he or she is going to be in your writing room all the time" (p. 220). Wilma Clark, thank you for being in my writing room all the time. You have helped me understand the big and little of writing—see "clunky-ness," use semicolons, integrate description (not too much and not too little), design a pace, weave in dialogue to spark the page, and move beyond abstraction to specific examples that speak to the reader. Ah, the reader. Most of all you have helped me see and honor the reader. Because your feedback is always direct, clear, explicit, and clothed in gentleness, I never once was tempted to bristle or counter with a "Yeah, but . . . " With your skill and with your grace, as a teacher and as a friend, Wilma, while I was writing this book you have been one of the people that mattered the most.

Thank you to Karen Witt, who is my treasured mentor–friend, and who helped me teach and learn from my wobbly beginnings. In helping me grow, the words attributed to Dinah Maria Craik suit you best: *Oh, the comfort, the inexpressible comfort of feeling safe with a person, having neither to weigh thought nor measure word, but pouring them all right out, just as they are, chaff and grain together, certain that a faithful hand will take and sift them, keep what is worth keeping, and with a breath of kindness, blow the rest away.* Karen, thank you for your dedicated and learned camaraderie.

Stephen Nowak, my father and my first teacher, helped me discover many things. I acknowledge here his hand in helping me seek and cherish the written word. When our biweekly milk check earned less than $4, he still subscribed to a daily newspaper. Even though it was a day late coming down our dusty gravel road, he harshly silenced all our noisy childish imp that distracted him while he read that newspaper every evening cover to cover. And on Sunday afternoons he would pull from the top pantry shelf the only hardcover book in our house, *American Wild Life Illustrated* (1955) so that we could all take turns comparing the blurry grey photos of the porcupine fish to the puffer fish. In it, too, we read with a mix of fright and delight the seven actions to take if bitten by a snake. I still have the book, signed in my father's bold hand; that same hand continues to caress my love of reading. *Dziękuję Tata.*

My mother, Josephine, was also a teacher. From her I learned strength and stubbornness, hardiness and common sense. Because of what she did, I learned to hear the voices of the silent, the vulnerable, the disabled, and the people on the bottom rungs of society's ladder. Most importantly, I learned from my mother that those voices must be cared for when everyone else slithers out of the room. Regardless of what she said to me, I also learned that deep inside she is proud of me and cares about my life. And now she rests in peace.

My brothers: Anthony, Wence, Simon, Wally, and Andy. Despite not knowing exactly what I was writing, your questions and your air of pride warmed me at the fire that is the quiet grit, the unpretentious survivorship, and the resilient solidarity of our family. For your rock-solid kindness over the years, especially during my dark days; for never expecting any return; and for always holding me tenderly in the glow of that Nowak campfire—I am forever thankful.

My sister, Jennie. How do people make it through life without a sister? In your captivating curiosity about all things new, you take me with you—watching the sandhill cranes from a blind lit by the early dawn of Kearney, Nebraska, or hosting Wayne and me at your teaching in the Democratic Republic of the Congo, or studying the history of Middle Eastern Muslim women, or reading McCullough's account of the building of the Panama Canal. It is your hunger and respect for discoveries such as these that have helped me learn about learning and write about teaching. And always, always, Jennie, you listen to me with compassion and speak to me with reason. For that I am grateful.

Thank you to my nephew Scott Petrack. You have filled my life with jest and joke, with humanity and helpfulness, with a nudge to practice patience and easiness, and with a spontaneity that will not quit—all the ways of the educator.

And my deepest gratitude and love to my husband, Wayne. I could list the million things you have done, opening with the morning mocha you made "expressly" to initiate ideas and ending with a happy hour to silence the day, and all the computer tasks, household chores, and life maintenance in between. There seems to be nothing you cannot do. Thank you, Wayne, for all of this. For a range of reasons, the 2 years of this book writing have not been simple or light for you. Yet—every single day, with unhurried intention and abundant love—you wrapped this book dream in a silken cloth and helped me bring it to the dawn.

REFERENCE

King, S. (2000). *On writing: A memoir of the craft.* New York: Pocket Books.

Knowing the Self as Teacher

CHAPTER 1

Then and Now: A Call to Pause

By three methods we may learn wisdom:
First, by reflection which is noblest;
Second, by imitation, which is the easiest; and
Third, by experience, which is the bitterest.

—Confucius

It all began with Cherry Ames: *Cherry Ames, Student Nurse*; *Cherry Ames, Senior Nurse*. In those fictional book series, she was the smart, passionate and beautiful, and lucky (albeit shallow) nurse with an attitude who charmed me and countless other young teenagers of the 1960s. Cherry Ames enticed us into the corridors and operating rooms of hospitals, enamored us with the thrill of learning facts and saving lives, and tempted us with the romance that blossomed in the dormitory tunnels and stairwells. During those unnerving Vietnam War years, the lure for me was the irresistible science of biology and physiology and my foggy fascination with literature, art history, and social studies. Along with thousands of other baby boomers, I was hooked.

LEARNING AND TEACHING

That was then; this is now.

In between were a baccalaureate nursing degree, years of acute care and critical care nursing, graduate degrees, and a venture into higher education, teaching first at a community college level and then at a university. Without a doubt, these alphabet soup adventures did not follow a precise plan; I floundered and flailed, bending as the breezes blew me. Incidentally, although it works for some, I find it difficult to suggest that a definite 1-, 5-, and 10-year career plan is essential.

Others may consider my career decisions uninformed, based on poor rationale, or even made under some duress. As part of the flounder and flail, I pursued a baccalaureate degree simply because Mr. Larry Stephenson, my

3

wise high school counselor, told me to. I had already selected a nearby diploma program because I marveled at the picture on its marketing brochure (perhaps it lured me in true Cherry Ames style). Instead, Mr. Stephenson convincingly handed me the application to the University of Wisconsin–Eau Claire, "Fill this out and mail it in by the end of the week." After this persuasion and too mortified to admit that I didn't even know where Eau Claire was located, I rushed home and gently unwrapped, so as not to further rip the creases, our 20-year-old ragged state map. Eau Claire, the "state's most beautiful campus," lay 200 miles directly west of my tiny hometown. Not surprisingly, I did not breathe a word about this to anyone at home. I was 17, from a rural impoverished family whose mother and father scarcely completed fourth and sixth grade and I hadn't a clue about higher education. Mr. Stephenson, please hear my thank-you!

After a few years of staff nursing, I entered a master's in nursing program at California State University–Los Angeles and focused on education. The tuition was minimal in California at the time and I thought I would have evenings, weekends, and holidays off as an instructor. I know, I know . . . I hear your chuckles and chortles—what was I thinking?

And then, more flounder. My decision to pursue doctoral education was delayed and fraught with hesitancy, self-doubt, and a lack of understanding about its value and career implications. The real truth is that I entered the PhD program at the University of Wisconsin–Milwaukee shaking and shivering. I felt like I was molded to the smallest space possible and I believed that I would never do anything that would take my own breath away.

Being a learner and a teacher has been my career—no, my life. After one year in an associate degree program, my faculty experience has been in baccalaureate and master's nursing education. For 30 years, I have taught and learned with students at all levels in the classroom and in clinical settings, and with various synchronous and asynchronous technical methods. The content areas that have most absorbed me are nursing care of adults in acute care, education, leadership, research, and international collaboration. Throughout most of my tenure as a nurse educator, I have integrated an active practice as a staff nurse and professional clinical consultant into my teaching and scholarship role.

That was then; this is now.

A MOMENT IN TIME

As they go on, the days plead for a pause. How have the years unfolded? Alice Walker, in her recent book *We Are the Ones We Have Been Waiting For*

(2006), admonishes us to pause, noting that the moment something major is accomplished, we are so relieved to finally be done with it, that we are already rushing into the future. Perhaps this accomplishment is completing a graduate degree, ending a semester, taking on a new position, or earning tenure. In one way or another, we always seem to be bolting forward. Wisdom, she suggests, exacts a pause and demands that we stop, sit down, and reflect in a universal place of rest to bask in the warmth of wonder.

I must tell you about my recent experience around "pause." I had the pleasure of co-teaching a doctoral course that focused on scholarly writing at Borås University College in Sweden with my cherished friend and colleague, Dr. Margret Lepp. As Margret and I planned each 6-hour day, she kept repeating, "We need to plan the time for a pause. . . . What are we going to do for the pause?"

At first I was confused about what she meant by using this word: *pause*. English was her second language; perhaps I misunderstood her meaning. But then, I finally got it. Margret meant that the class needed to take a break—we needed to plan for the class break.

Then, I must admit, my nasty ethnocentrism kicked in. I thought, how quaint, how "off" to use the term *pause* inaccurately in this way. I supposed this was similar to Margret using the word *sprinkles* when she meant *freckles*, or when she said we needed to get "installed" in our hotel room when she meant "check in." "Pause," I self-righteously chuckled to myself with a dose of smug.

But the more I thought about *pause*, the more suitable the term seemed. It reveals more than the class taking a break. *Break* implies broken and fractured, sounds pinched and creased. Just as Margret and I paused in our teaching and learning through the day, the class also paused, all to breathe with a sigh of curiosity and conjecture and warmth. This experience was one of a hundred like it where Margret helped me see, helped me pause to explore another moment in time.

PAUSES AT DEPARTURE AND ARRIVAL

Pauses are fundamental especially when we gingerly edge into a new place, pass over yet another threshold, move into nursing education. Thresholds are sacred turning points—they mark the place where what is ending has not yet transformed into that which is about to be. Thresholds are the in-between spaces, the aerial gap flanked by two trapeze bars. As Amy Tan (2005) alleges, "to leave one place is not the same as entering another" (p. 141).

I thought about thresholds when I vacationed in Key West, Florida, and witnessed the partying that happens on the beach at sunset. Everyone heads to the beach in the late afternoon. As the sun slowly sinks and colors caress the edge of sky, the party noise cranks up, notch by notch. But during the few minutes when the sun nudges the horizon, everything silences and everyone turns to the sinking sun. This is the threshold moment—the crossing place from day to night—and it beckons us. People stop moving and talking and singing and dancing to be present as the sun melts into the sea.

Pausing in this way demands self-reflection; it is the chronic restlessness luring us forward at departures and arrivals. It helps us "mind the gap" as we seize the next trapeze bar.

Pausing to self-reflect is pilgrimage. Yet *pilgrimage* is different from *journey*. We often use *journey* as a metaphor for moving, growing, developing. Journey includes longing, getting ready, setting out, experiencing doubt and hope. Journey symbolizes drawing near or anticipation and arrival.

Pilgrimage is all that, too: longing, getting ready, setting out, experiencing doubt and hope, drawing near, or anticipation and arriving. But pilgrimage is also "coming home," coming back for reflection and redirection. As pilgrims, we place ourselves at risk.

First, a pilgrim does not return as the same person who set out. All that we think we know, all that we think we understand, all that we carefully plan and construct may be blown apart. Asking principal questions about who we are is risky, and we may learn things that we can't foresee. Who we are, our soul life is always greater the more we come to know it. Parker Palmer (2004) cautions us that exploring our "soul truth" must be done "on the slant" because it is so powerful. He submits that "third things" are helpful in this slant approach. The third things can be a piece of art, for example, that opens the door to personal expression, that may "invite, not command, the soul to speak . . . giving the shy soul the protective cover it needs" (pp. 92–93). Third things can be writing, weaving, or walking—things that invite and take us gently inward and downward.

Second, on a pilgrimage there is a risk that we will be surprised by joy. We encounter people, places, thoughts, feelings, visions, and happenings that take us beyond anything we might imagine. And certainly, when we come home—when we reflect and redirect—we are never the same again.

Most of us probably do not make the world-renowned pilgrimages to Mecca, Canterbury in England, or Chaco Canyon in New Mexico, or do not participate in the Home Dance of the Hopi Indians. But the inner pilgrimage beckons all of us—the honorable pilgrimage that both changes and surprises us.

YOU ARE YOURSELF

In our pilgrimage, in our self-reflection, we clarify who we are. We cannot look only to our role models, our heroes and heroines who have been "perfect" teachers for us, and strive to imitate them. Picasso described this effort at emulation: "You should constantly try to paint like someone else. But the thing is, you can't! You would like to. You try. But it turns out to be a botch. . . . And it's at the very moment you make a botch of it that you're yourself" (Parmelin, n.d., p. 43).

Imagine being a poet and attempting to write like William Butler Yeats, Robert Frost, or Emily Dickinson. Someone once said of Yeats: *Proud Ireland hurt you into poetry.* In all probability, these poets had a specific event or experience, their own place or unique life that "hurt them" into poetry. We hear and feel their own textures when we read them. The relaxed and conversational voice of Frost is distinct from the spare and mysterious voice of Dickinson. They ask us fiercely, as we put our poet pen to paper, "What has hurt *you* into poetry?"

In the same way, we must ask ourselves in our own self-reflection, What has hurt me into nursing education? What assets do I have? Precisely, who we are and what we have are the only places we can begin.

Being clear about who we are and what we have brings me back to a recent flipside opinion essay written by a savvy 20-something journalist. Like many communities, the Midwest city I live in is struggling to enhance its culture and entertainment life. Questions about what will charm people to visit or relocate to our city always dictate the discussion.

Instead, this astute journalist challenged city leaders to analyze what the *community residents* wanted and needed to make life better, rather than trying to predict what would make outsiders drool. He shrewdly maintained that if the residents were happy and engaged in a good life—their culture and entertainment life—outsiders would quickly notice and flock to the city. It was the city itself and the people living in it that are the center, not how many water parks are close to the interstate or how many chain restaurants string along the traffic routes. Heeding the journalist's counsel, then, we also must reflect on who we are and how we paint, and not be shallowly enticed by the "interstate water parks" in nursing education.

Admittedly, there is a shadow side to the pause, to self-reflection. Walker (2006) concedes that there may be a certain fear in pausing. Some of us may think that a pause has nothing in it, feels empty, or is worthless. Often we may see no end to it; we may not even see a beginning or a need for it. As a culture, we may not be in the habit of respecting, honoring, or even acknowledging the pause. There is a rush to act, the distaste for hesitation, the absolute hatred for spending time in emptiness.

Carol Shields (2002) describes the dark silhouette of pause in *Unless*, a novel about Reta Winters, a fiction writer whose daughter plummets into an emotional crisis. Reta says that "ordering my own house calms me down, my careful dusting, my polishing. Speculating about other people's lives helps, too . . . tricking the neural synapses into a grand avoidance of my own sorrow. The examined life has had altogether too much publicity. Introversion is piercingly dull in its circularity and lack of air" (p. 107).

Yet, we must respect and honor the pause though doing this may stifle, even suffocate us. We must plan a time for a pause in nursing higher education: to reflect and wonder; to explain, reconsider, and compromise; to lie fallow for a time; and to perhaps apologize and retreat. This pause demands that we stop our careful dusting and our polishing. A place to begin may be to peel back the layers of what we are dusting and why we are polishing. Whose house, after all, are we ordering?

In pausing to check on the house, to wonder in our pilgrimage, we realize the challenge of education is no longer purely intellectual, but rather in figuring out who we are. The process of becoming a teacher never seems quite complete. I'm always taken aback when I tell others that I'm a nurse educator. I yearn to ask myself: "You're a nurse educator already?" Sometimes I even feel a charlatan, holding my breath lest anyone probe further. We must work at having a clear image of ourselves, to not see and shape ourselves through other people's eyes. We must move, even if only in our minds, knowing perfectly well that when we dare ask the core questions about who we are we cannot predict all that will happen.

Albert Einstein connected wonder, the mystery of who we are, with emotion. Perhaps we don't often associate Einstein with feelings, but he wrote, "The most beautiful thing we can experience is the mysterious. It is the source of all true art and science. He to whom this emotion is a stranger, who can no longer pause to wonder and stand rapt in awe, is as good as dead: his eyes are closed. . . . To know that what is impenetrable to us really exists, manifesting itself as the highest wisdom and the most radiant beauty which our dull faculties can comprehend only in their most primitive forms" (Einstein, 1931, p. 6).

The integrity of who we are is distinctively described by Siamak, one of Moaveni's Iranian friends in her book *Lipstick Jihad* (2005). Siamak was using his experience with his forest-green Mustang convertible to discuss the "foolish idea that they (Iranian religious/political leaders) could take a Western concept, like democracy, alter it with Islamic attitudes toward women, and expect it to function properly." For his "Mustang therapy," as he called it,

Siamak cranked up Led Zeppelin and raced that antique ragtop around the streets of Tehran. To keep his Mustang running, the Iranian mechanic kept tinkering with it repeatedly, adding old Iranian parts, and then was shocked because it didn't work. To illustrate his point about integrity and authenticity, Siamak concludes, "It's the same with our politicians and intellectuals . . . they borrow Western concepts like democracy, stick in Iranian parts, and can't figure out why they've lost the juice" (p. 77).

In this pause, then, I must spend time with who I am. Who am I, without any parts added that don't belong, without mixing and affixing in ways that don't fit?

I must ask, who am I, not only what do I do? What I do is "doing education," that doing that breaks down teaching into shards and splinters: what we teach and perhaps how we teach. "Doing education" is when we think we teach only during our class time on Monday, Wednesday, Friday at 1 to 3 p.m. "Doing education" does not follow us home, insinuate into our evenings, and shade our thoughts as Maggie Jones did in Vaneta Masson's poem (Masson, 1991, pp. 56–60). Maggie Jones was the feisty and spirited woman of inner-city Washington, DC, who, as a patient, "followed" the nurse–poet home and affected Masson's daily life. When we merely "do education," then it does not follow us home.

Pausing at this threshold into nursing education, as we depart and arrive, means asking again in a multilayered and deeper way: Who was the Cherry Ames for you? Even though now she is described as a "porcelain-skinned, and vapid fictional nurse heroine . . . cultural equivalent of the Barbie doll" (Gorman, 2005, p. 90), the pause demands that we remember what hurt us into nursing, and then tempted us further into nursing education.

In pausing to remember then and now, in learning wisdom, the noble rituals of reflection invite the soul to speak and memorialize who you are. And then, how have the years unfolded through your practice and education? Focusing on who you are, not what you do, challenges you to ask what is right with you (not what is wrong with you). In this way, on the slant, you will see the beauty Einstein assured would reach us only indirectly.

REFERENCES

Einstein, A. (1931). *Living philosophies: A series of intimate credos.* New York: Simon and Schuster.

Gorman, G. (2005). So long, Cherry Ames. *American Journal of Nursing, 105*(2), 90–92.

Masson, V. (1999). *Rehab at the Florida Avenue Grill.* Washington, DC: Sage Femme Press.

Moaveni, A. (2005). *Lipstick jihad: A memoir of growing up Iranian in America and American in Iran.* New York: PublicAffairs of the Perseus Books Group.

Palmer, P. J. (2004). *A hidden wholeness: The journey toward an undivided life.* San Francisco: Jossey-Bass Publishers.

Parmelin, H. (n.d.). *Picasso: The artist and his model and other recent works.* New York: Harry N. Abrams.

Shields, C. (2002). *Unless.* New York: HarperCollins Publishers.

Tan, A. (2005). *Saving fish from drowning.* New York: Ballantine Books.

Walker, A. (2006). *We are the ones we have been waiting for: Inner light in a time of darkness.* New York: The New Press.

CHAPTER 2

Honoring the Present in the Best and Worst Year

It is best to learn as we go, not go as we have learned.

—Leslie Jeanne Sahler

Melissa was completing her master's degree in nursing with an emphasis on education. During her final year of graduate school, she also held her first faculty position teaching nursing full-time. In a written reflection at the end of that year, Melissa examined her experience in an essay titled "The Best and Worst Year."

That year began in a late summer phone conversation in which she was offered a teaching position for the fall term. Her hiring supervisor told Melissa that the first year would be "icky . . . this is to be expected . . . the icky-ness . . . things would get better after the first year."

After accepting the position and hanging up the phone, Melissa puzzled frantically about "icky," as her rising pulse and tightening breath jammed her throat. The start date was clear, the employment benefits were expected, the teaching assignment was explicit (albeit a bit daunting)—but icky? In her essay, Melissa wrote, "Why would it be icky? Would this job consume my time, would I not know what to do, would no one help me?" In her end-of-the-year essay, she untangled the threads of icky-ness—what they were and how she survived.

Because of her current acute care clinical expertise, Melissa generally felt comfortable with the clinical teaching responsibilities. But, as the start date neared, her anxiety about classroom and skills lab teaching escalated miserably, nearly reaching out-and-out despair. In fact, Melissa wondered if she could still be released from the contract: "I found myself wishing for a car accident to get me out of the first semester. I thought a broken leg would probably be sufficient injury to buy me a little time."

As Melissa's year unfolded, she began to understand her supervisor's admonitions. Unfamiliarity with the course and semester flow, untried learning

11

activities in the course, and little skill in planning how the time would be used in the classroom all loomed insurmountable. Written midsemester feedback from students multiplied her anxiety; one student wrote that if Melissa were to "lighten up a little, they were sure she would be a fun person." (I wonder if these same students in their first clinical contact with real patients were able to "lighten up"? But that is another essay.)

Then, the second semester presented a grueling new course to teach. Melissa barely remembered Wilms's tumor or open-angle glaucoma or cardiac muscle action potentials from her own nursing education. And now she was expected to be the expert in these areas, to teach creatively, even to write valid and reliable multiple-choice test items.

On good days, Melissa mused, "Where was that car accident or broken leg when you most needed it?" All in all, employment as a new faculty, finishing graduate school, and home and relationship responsibilities merged to make it her best and worst year.

QUARRYING THE FIRST-YEAR CHALLENGES

With perceptive tenderness and buoyancy, Melissa described her first year angst as a nurse educator and recounted survival. As I read her candid reflections, I recalled countless mentoring and precepting conversations I've had with other new faculty in their first year. One novice nurse educator, with no formal preparation in teaching or curriculum and program development, recently confessed that "at first I believed I could learn it 'on the job,' but it does not seem too realistic now." And of course I easily summon up my own clumsy-stumbly first years. Please know that I'm using *the first year* as a symbolic phrase. Even though in reality the time might be a semester, a year, or two or three, "the first year" is our time as beginners, as neophytes, as novices. Time and again, I'm reminded how familiar, and yet disturbing, awkward, uncertain, and painful, our first year can be.

The awkwardness and naiveté (but also the conviction and resilience) of the first teaching experience are akin to Dennis the Menace's retort to Margaret when she notices he's reading a book upside down. Margaret charges him with her usual gloat, "Face it, Dennis, you've got a long way to go in the Education Department."

Dennis does not flinch in his haughtiness, "That's what you think . . . all I gotta do is get through next year."

Margaret noses closer, with her pointed finger and tilted hip, "And what are you going to do with a first grade education?"

Dennis smugly proclaims, "Teach Kindergarten!"

Like Dennis, I held books upside down (figuratively, and perhaps literally). And as a rule I shuffled only one small step ahead of the students—teaching kindergarten as a bumbling first grader.

Our experiences in the first several years of teaching have been well documented in the research (Anibas, Hanson Brenner, & Zorn, in press; Lewallen, Crane, Letvak, Jones, & Hu, 2003; Siler & Kleiner, 2001; Solem & Foote, 2004). In these studies, new educators faced countless challenges: considerable coursework requiring extensive preparation time; committee demands; balancing employment and home responsibilities; and insecurity about classroom and clinical teaching methods and student evaluation strategies.

In one of the studies (Anibas et al., in press), feelings of novice teaching academic staff was one of five major categories that emerged from the data. In that study, 10 participants from three baccalaureate nursing programs were interviewed about their experiences as new nurse educators. They described frustration, isolation, expendability, uncertainty about their own performance, and fear about patient and student safety.

In this research (Anibas et al., in press) one participant stated, "That was the part that was a little scary, just not knowing exactly what to expect . . . especially setting limits . . . being younger . . . you wonder if you're going to get that respect from students." Other individuals in that study described their stress in the following ways: "I felt really nervous and that was a really big stressor to me that I wasn't familiar with this hospital" and "I was really really worried that with the senior students that they would know more than I did." Finally, one research participant referred to PhD-prepared faculty in the setting, "I feel that distinction, not on the level that a PhD thinks they are better than you . . . just you're an expendable part of this university" and "if somebody with a PhD comes along that our job is gone."

Dr. Lee Shulman (2004), an internationally acclaimed teacher–leader and one of my very favorite authors, also examined what it is to be a new educator. What are some of the challenges that new teachers are tackling? In comparing experienced teachers to new teachers, those who were well practiced could tell what students don't understand, the concepts or ideas that frequently confuse the learner, and the mistaken perceptions that persist. Experienced teachers have figured most of that out and can work with it as they teach.

In contrast to the experienced teachers, new teachers frequently could not identify what pieces of content or perspectives the students would find challenging, or what flawed insights or views the students brought to their learning. New teachers had to work diligently to discover that, and it often took several classes or semesters to become "tuned in" to some of the students' thinking. In other words, the new educator must be educated.

Teaching the research process with beginning nursing students in my first years illustrates the comparison between new and experienced teachers. The students easily understood protecting the rights of research participants that, of course, is similar to confidentiality in nurse–patient communication (which they were learning concurrently). I probably spent more time than necessary with the participants' rights content; no wonder the students thought it a bit dry and dreary.

At the same time, these students found the research designs content almost unmanageable. It took me several semesters to learn about the students' difficulty with designs and, only then, did I begin to use multiple examples to "play with" this content. Previously, I assumed it was the students' problem—they just weren't getting it, not studying carefully, not reading the extremely detailed 42-page chapter on research designs.

To be truthful, I suspect that at that time I also understood the participants' rights content more clearly than I understood research designs. Hence, I probably spent more class time on this content because I knew it better.

My experience has been supported by research: The more familiar we are with the content, the more examples we use. In one study, Shulman (2004) noted a salient difference between two groups of teachers and their ability to illustrate and clarify with examples. Physics teachers explained the physics content using a wide array of examples, analogies, and metaphors; they were able to come at the content from multiple perspectives. But when biology teachers were teaching physics, they were limited to one example and "then they just died."

I have "just died" many times. Since those early years, I still have this balance problem. Even now I frequently emphasize content that I know with more examples, more class time, more learning activities, and more fun—regardless of the content's significance or how clearly and easily students understand it. For me, balancing content areas necessitates constant vigilance.

As we begin teaching (especially if the content is less familiar to us), maybe we also have too few examples at our fingertips. In preparing for class, I intentionally jot a brief phrase that reminds me of an example throughout my lecture notes; in fact, I plan many more examples than I usually use. They come from my nursing practice, my own experiences as a patient or family member, or I just make them up. When I began teaching I thought that I could recall or make up examples in class on the spot. I never acquired that skill, so I methodically and thoroughly plan ahead. As I've gained more experience, I'm able to use a student's encounter or question from earlier in the class period or from a previous class meeting and shape or revise it to fit a new idea that we're discussing and I store these examples for future classes.

Here are some examples of examples that have worked for me. My inaccurate use of random sampling in a statewide-study of RNs illustrates sampling methods. My misinterpretation of an insulin order helps review insulin types, transcribing orders, and medication error follow-up. I also share with students the time I recommended milk of magnesia to a patient with chronic kidney disease (and the resulting backlash); the students remember the mineral and electrolyte changes with renal pathology more easily. By the way, I also do have some examples that were not muddles on my part.

Another way to generate an example is to incorporate recent newspaper articles reporting the latest health study. I've drawn on "Broccoli Cures Uterine Cancer in Mice," "Echinacea Prevents Colds in Schoolchildren," and "Cardiac Patients Benefit from a Daily Beer." Not only can this type of example be used to review the pathophysiology and interventions, but research methods, journalism's role and responsibility, literature appraisal, and a broad spectrum of patient education issues can also be analyzed.

For the new nurse faculty, then, growth means learning about the self and the nursing students at the outset, reviewing the depth and breadth of specific content, and discovering how the students meet the content. It is this learning, reviewing, and discovering that is taking me a lifetime to master. Like Dennis, sometimes I still hold the book upside down, but I am always fortified by his determined "all I gotta do is get through next year."

HONORING THE PRESENT AND RENEWING ITS NOBILITY

In getting through next year, honoring the present and renewing its nobility offer a resource for those months or years as a novice. Examining, respecting, and valuing our own learning process are keys in this honoring and renewal of nobility. Too often, we may expect perfection or even feel shameful in our learning.

When we honor the present and renew its nobility, we cherish how we learn as teachers and how we develop as educators. Honoring the present is a way of thinking; it is making room for the essentials of who we are. It is living and experiencing rather than controlling or solving.

There seems to be a paradox in honoring and thinking about the present. The Chinese character for *person* depicts a figure grounded in the earth and stretching toward heaven. Why so seemingly becalmed on one end, yet so relentlessly restless on the other? This Chinese character suggests the destiny of every human being: to be fated, but also to be free—to be both free and fated.

Each of us is planted in the mud and the muck of daily existence, thrust into a world not of our choosing, and tethered then and there to hard-rock reality. Yet, equally so, and this is the paradox, we are also endowed with a mind able to reflect on that reality, to be mindful, to choose how to be in light of the cold facts. Melissa depicted the mud and muck of her best and worst year, as well as the reflective mindfulness that sustained her. In the ability to live that paradox lie the honor and the nobility.

Like the Chinese character for person that shows us both calm and restlessness, the mountains too show us fate, on the one hand, but also the freedom on the other. There is the humdrum daily-ness, rooted in rock, surviving the fog, rain, snow, and cold of the mountain base. But there is also the loftiness, stature, and freedom of the mountain tops—the height that helps us reflect, live, and treasure the aesthetic "now."

Twisting this idea a bit differently, the new nurse educator most typically joins a new employing organization. On the one hand, the new faculty quickly becomes rooted and tethered by policy and procedure, by evaluation criteria, perhaps by tenure prospects (or at least is expected to). The word *obligation* comes to mind. On the other hand, the autonomy required to be an effective teacher is essential. This autonomy can come easily, be granted freely in some settings, but it also may require delicate hewing, on the slant, in other settings.

Merging autonomy and obligation, which can sometimes be incompatible viewpoints, makes for a delicate, sometimes edgy position—another paradox. I've discovered that settling a little closer to the margin of both viewpoints makes for more flexibility and negotiation, more opportunity and possibility, rather than fixing stolidly in the center of one or the other. When living on the margin, one can move back and forth between obligation and autonomy more easily. Ideally, of course, organization and policy create the frame within which the professional can easily make good decisions according to best practice.

I was recently discussing the idea of paradox, of tether and freedom, with my friend Namji, who is an exquisite concert pianist and Korean by ethnic background. She instantly connected with the mountain analogy, of being fated and being free. "It's like music," Namji said. "Music is written . . . it is the fate. But as a performing musician, I am free to interpret it. I live the music. My performance of the written music is always very different than someone else's performance of it. And my performance of the same piece of music is different every time I play it . . . and that is my freedom."

As a new educator, then, how does one honor the present and renew its nobility? How do we live the music, perform the same piece differently every time? What are the loftiness and stature, the freedom of being a novice teacher?

WHERE HAVE I BEEN AS TEACHER?

Being rooted in a true sense of self underpins the freedom of being teacher. In fact, recognizing who we are intensifies our capacity to do good work. Parker Palmer, in his landmark book *The Courage to Teach* (1998) raises the question about who is the self that teaches, maintaining that this exploration of who we are "honors and challenges the teacher's heart, and it invites a deeper inquiry than our traditional questions" (p. 4).

Customarily, according to Palmer, we first ask the "what" question. As new faculty we may fret about the amount of detail we "must" include in our lecture on septic shock or how many theories of aging the students "must" know. Often, we stop at the "what" questions. But in deepening the conversation, we may ask the "how" questions—how do students learn best about global health or how research can be used to guide nursing practice. Perhaps occasionally, but probably rarely, as new educators do we ask the "why" question; that is, for what purpose do we teach? And seldom if ever, Palmer asserts, do we ask the "who" question—who is the self that teaches? How does who I am shape how I relate to the students, the content, my colleagues, and the bigger world?

Asking about who is the self that teaches honors the present of who we are as new faculty. How does our previous experience as students or our own practice as nurses form or deform who we are as teachers? How do our lives as citizens mold who we are as teachers?

Evolving as a teacher, I stepped from one wet rocky stone to another, slipping and clutching as I went along. My own ability to honor the present, to contemplate the self as an educator, was cultivated over time and now continually extends.

Initially, I saw myself as the focal point—how did I appear to the students? Would the students like me? Even, what did the students think about the clothes I was wearing or my hairstyle? Was I viewed as knowledgeable? As the students posed question after question, demanding instant answers, I expected myself to provide answer after answer immediately. I certainly could not listen to my inner voice saying "wait" and "listen." I did not have the wisdom to withhold, to support learning rather than teaching as the priority process. Admittedly, this focus was on the self, but at a shallow surface level.

After embracing the spotlight with my concern about being liked and looking smart, I then concentrated on the students. I remember being extensively concerned about each of them, their personal lives, out-of-class activities, family, and friends. I socialized with many of them. I challenged myself to memorize as many details as possible about all of their lives.

Shortly after this focus on students, I emphasized the depth and detail of the content I was teaching. I tried to learn everything possible about the specific subject matter and fully expected all the students to have that same depth and breadth of understanding. I was a skilled clinician and insisted that the students entering the profession should be experts as well. After all, every student should be a specialist in the most advanced cardiac monitoring and intervention, right? Obviously, I was honoring neither the students' present nor my own.

So, in more deeply examining who am I who teaches, I moved from a superficial focus on self to perhaps an excessive, unnecessary connection with students to content overkill. In a few situations, these emphases may have been beneficial, perhaps even temporarily rich and meaningful. But overall, I've learned that none of these "places" was useful in the long term because they were not a part of a centeredness that was me as teacher. At times, I felt deceitful, almost a sham. These places eroded the freedom to examine the self, honor the present, and renew its nobility.

WHERE AM I GOING AS TEACHER?

Part of the centeredness that is me as teacher requires that I examine where I am going. As I help other novice educators with classroom and clinical teaching, the art and the impact of posing questions with students frequently surfaces. I must concede my own need for some remodeling.

First, perhaps because of my impatience or my desire to "tell what I know," or my discomfort with silence, I often respond to my own questions much too quickly. I have found this to be true with other educators as well (both novice and veteran teachers). Responding too quickly to one's own question tends to end the discussion because the students then perceive the teacher as the expert.

Again, borrowing from Lee Shulman's (2004) discussion, I'd like to highlight some notions about wait times, the amount of time between a teacher's question and a student's response. As supported by research, when teachers wait longer to get a student response or before they repeated, restated, or redirected the question, student responses are more complex, analytic, and creative. Incidentally, the wait times in the research were extended from the average 1 second to what Shulman identifies as "a veritable pedagogical eternity" (about 4 seconds) (p. 262).

There is an additional research finding particularly relevant to the novice teacher. Longer wait times result in more student responses that were unpredictable; that is, the teacher didn't expect what the student said and may not be able to quickly discern whether the response is "right or wrong." Shulman (2004) describes this phenomenon as putting "the greatest strain on the subject-matter competence of the teacher, who now had to delve into his or her understanding . . . to think of a way of coping with this strange, or at least unexpected, response" (p. 263). Thus, perhaps we keep our wait times short (closer to 1 second) when we are less experienced or teaching unfamiliar content to safeguard our credibility and expose less of our self as teacher.

Waiting and listening before we respond with an answer or a question are critical, but doing so can be grueling, especially if we're in unfamiliar territory. First, waiting feels like infinity and, second, waiting may result in student responses that stagger and render us speechless.

If higher-level cognitive responses are a goal and longer wait times help facilitate them, how might we manage some of the unease associated with longer wait times? I've always meant to videotape a class or two that I'm teaching, and then actually measure my wait times and appraise the students' responses. This would be another way to know the self as teacher, perhaps with stunning results. I've purposely practiced extending wait times, which has become more comfortable for me. I've also practiced some responses to student's comments when I'm walking on tentative ground: "I'm not sure exactly, but my guess is that . . ." or "I don't know, but an important idea that closely relates to your question is . . ." or "I don't know for certain, but what do others think about this question?" (then more wait time) or "I'm not sure, but let me try to see what I can learn about it and get back to you." Then, I always make every effort to return publicly with a response: "Last week Eric asked about . . . What I found is that . . ." This, of course, affirms Eric and his question, invites more questions from everyone, and reveals my continued sense of inquiry.

In addition to considering wait times and their influence on higher-level thinking, the teacher also must take time to word questions carefully. Frequently, usually without even thinking, a yes/no question or a vague opener may be posed. For example, in an attempt to encourage reflection after viewing a video about gender differences in communication, the teacher might ask, "Do you see similarities between the video and the communication on your nursing unit?" or "Did you see your own style of talking illustrated in the video?" Or, in a post-clinical conference, the clinical instructor might ask, "So how was your day?" The result in these situations is head-nodding all around, "fine," or "okay."

Taking time to word questions carefully is essential. I suggest that teachers plan and write down questions ahead of time that encourage students to synthesize information, draw conclusions, and apply concepts to practice. Without preplanning and prewriting, often the teacher falls back on the comfortable, easy yes/no or simple fact query and does not go further.

Returning to the video about gender differences in communication, the teacher may begin with a *concrete* question where students are asked to recall information: "What were the three major gender differences discussed?" or "What childhood experiences contribute to the gender differences in communication?" A concrete question in postclinical conference might be, "What are the common analgesics used with the postsurgical patients on this unit and what side effects are you anticipating?" Concrete questions may be used to get started, set the groundwork, put facts out on the table.

An *abstract* question then encourages higher level thinking by requiring the student to classify or draw conclusions. For example, "How are the gender differences in the video similar to or different from the discussion in Chapter 6 in your book?" or "In your work in the public health department over the last 5 weeks, what gender differences in communication have you noticed in the nurse–client relationship? Which approach suggested in the video might be most effective in these situations and why?" Abstract questions may also examine reasons and evidence ("What evidence supports your perspective about this?"), probe other viewpoints ("How might other groups of students respond?"), and identify consequences ("What might happen if this was done?").

As I go forward as teacher, I want to keep the art and impact of posing questions continually on my radar screen. For me, several "must remembers" plead for attention: (1) word the question distinctively, without vague phrases or embedded in general discussion, (2) summarize the students' responses to affirm their thinking and repeat key ideas, (3) invite other students to elaborate (this moves discussion from only student–teacher interaction to student–student interaction), and (4) avoid "grilling" where the teacher bombards with multiple questions in sequence or poses a block of questions at once.

THE EDUCATOR MOVES INSIDE

The freedom to know the self as teacher is held up by our mindfulness as we question our view of the world and our place in it. *Mindfulness* means paying particular attention in a particular way, on purpose, in the present, and nonjudgmentally. It is a way to get back in touch with our own wisdom and vitality, focus inwardly and deliberately, and take charge of the direction and quality of our own lives.

In my own mindfulness, in paying attention to becoming who I am as educator, I've realized that *educator* has moved from the outside to my inside. I think this is happening because I've opened myself for *educator* to shape me, to move inside. When *educator* was outside, the focus was on me, as the shallow self, as well as the social connections with students and the piles of content. As the educator is moving inside, I'm appreciating that education is really all three: me, the students, and the content. Actually, it is the relationship among all three that is education.

Annie Dillard (1989) describes this internalizing process happening in working-class France. In that situation, when an apprentice was injured or got tired, the experienced workers said, "It is the trade entering his body" (p. 69). Dillard also describes art and the painter in this way. The painter does not use paint to control or glue down the world—the tubes of paint become the fingers as the brain changes physical shape to fit the paint.

Perhaps *education* must enter our body also, to become our thoughts and actions, beginning in the gritty and frothy first year. When it is outside, we may attempt to fasten the students, mournfully mold them. It may be that, initially, we try to fit the discipline, the classroom, the world to ourselves. As *educator* enters us, then, we must fit ourselves to education, recognizing that as this happens, we cannot hurry and we cannot rest.

Shulman (2004) describes Charles Bosk's book *Forgive and Remember*, about surgical interns learning in their residency, to support using cases as a pedagogical tool. In analyzing cases with students, according to Shulman, we can begin to learn from the case experience, rather than to focus on counting failures and hiding embarrassment.

In a similar way, as the book title indicates, errors will be made (no, must be made) as we learn to be educators, as educator enters us. Draped and croaky skeletons loitering in all our educator closets plead to be forgiven and remembered. I have a skeleton that frequently gnaws at me about my early efforts at cooperative learning. *Cooperative learning* is a group method built on interdependence, relationship, and accountability, among other characteristics. After attending a 2-day conference fully geared toward K through 12 education (I was the only university educator in an audience of more than 300 primary and secondary teachers), I came back an out-and-out convert to cooperative learning, albeit a blundering amateur. In my uninformed fervor, I even had the university students in my class raising their hands to signal "quiet time."

It wasn't until one of the students gently enlightened me, "You're treating us like children," that I stepped back and reassessed. Things were just not working. Several factors contributed to my ineptness: (1) I didn't apply cooperative learning to the students in *my* classroom—I merely applied a canned approach to which I was briefly exposed, (2) I didn't seek help from a colleague along the way, discussing the process and struggles as I went along, and (3) I didn't examine how cooperative learning fit with me, my style, my philosophy of education. As with all of our educator skeletons, honoring the present insists that we forgive and remember—reflect, celebrate, and learn from that entering experience.

I'd like to return to Melissa as she honored the present by forgiving and remembering in her "Best and Worst Year" essay. As her "educator" moved from the outside to the inside in that novice teaching experience, several lessons surfaced. First, anxiety is a given. No matter what educational preparation one has, or how many hours one prepares for a lecture, or how many textbooks on basic skills one pours over, Melissa notes that "I am not sure if I would have felt any more confident that first day." She also recognizes that a teacher must live through a course at least one time to help the students navigate it: "it was really hard for me to explain to the students the flow of the semester and the assignments when I really had very little understanding of how things would go."

Student evaluations were an additional source of anxiety for Melissa. Initially, she was "heartbroken when I read some of the things" even recalling that "for the rest of the semester every time I went to class, I was thinking 'someone out there thinks I do not know what I am doing; someone out there thinks I do not have any fun while I am here.' " Yet, and this is Bosk's "forgiving and remembering," Melissa had the courage to thank students for their feedback, learn from the comments, and carry on with the course.

Despite Melissa's angst, as her educator moved inside, she felt some self-confidence, trusted that she could improve, and knew that "I had potential. . . . I am a work in progress." With practice and help from others, the educator was shaped.

What form did "help from others" take? Melissa clearly declares several sources: (1) specific family members, (2) teaching colleagues, (3) graduate student colleagues and classes, and (4) readings, particularly Albom's *Tuesdays with Morrie*, Ayers' *Teaching Toward Freedom*, and Palmer's *Courage to Teach*.

In her essay's final paragraph, Melissa convinces: "It is okay to be a novice. This is who I am at this point in my life. Why should I hide from this when I could instead be embracing who I am?" This self-assurance is echoed by David Whyte (1994), a poet who has used his creativity to preserve the soul of corporate America. He distinguishes between our "wish to have power *over* experience, to control all events and consequences, and the soul's wish to have power *through* experience" (p. 17). Melissa gained power through her experiences.

Mindfulness, then, invites us to grow and learn *through* the novice experience; learning requires that we rearrange isolated work events into the experience of self as teacher. These isolated work events—the routine, the daily-ness—are "the drab of grit that seeps into an oyster's shell that makes the pearl, not pearl-making seminars with other oysters" (King, 2000, p. 235). We grow as nurse educators, then, primarily because we experience and reflect on our novicehood, not because we attend education conferences.

Honoring the present requires the Zen master's "beginner's mind," the eagerness to look at the world as if for the first time. Honoring the present demands that we step out of the learning process and see it fresh once more. It is in that stepping out, learning as we go (not going as we have learned) that we emerge blinking and stunned with the *educator* inside.

REFERENCES

Anibas, M., Hanson Brenner, G., & Zorn C. R. (In press). Experiences described by novice teaching academic staff (TAS) in baccalaureate nursing education: A focus on mentoring. *Journal of Professional Nursing.*

Dillard, A. (1989). *The writing life.* New York: HarperCollins Publishers.

King, S. (2000). *On writing: A memoir of the craft.* New York: Pocket Books.

Lewallen, L. P., Crane, P. B., Letvak, S., Jones, E., & Hu, J. (2003). An innovative strategy to enhance new faculty success. *Nursing Education Perspectives, 24*(5), 257–260.

Palmer, P. J. (1998). *The courage to teach: Exploring the inner landscape of a teacher's life.* San Francisco: Jossey-Bass Publishers.

Shulman, L. S. (2004). *The wisdom of practice: Essays on teaching, learning, and learning to teach.* San Francisco: Jossey-Bass Publishers.

Siler, B., & Kleiner, C. (2001). Novice faculty: Encountering expectations in academia. *Journal of Nursing Education, 40*(9), 397–403.

Solem, M., & Foote, K. (2004). Concerns, attitudes, and abilities of early-career geography faculty. *Annals of the Association of American Geographers, 94*(4), 889–912.

Whyte, D. (1994). *The heart aroused: Poetry and the preservation of the soul in corporate America.* New York: Doubleday.

CHAPTER 3

"As If": More of That First Year

Learning from experience is a faculty almost never practiced.

—Barbara Tuchman

"As if" emerges persuasively in the first year of teaching. Until recently, "as if" seemed just another handy phrase, but now I see its convincing command penetrate the new nurse educator's launch into the faculty role.

Several authors credit the might and muscle of others to their "as if" posture. For example, in *Lipstick Jihad*, Azadeh Moaveni (2005) describes how Iran's young generation is changing that nation "from below." In their "as if" lifestyle, the people born just before or along with the revolution "act 'as if' it was permitted to hold hands on the street, blast music at parties, speak your mind, challenge authority, take your drug of choice, grow your hair long, wear too much lipstick . . . they will decide Iran's future" (p. ix). Similarly, Hitchens (2001) honors Vaclav Havel who lived "as if" in a free society, Aleksandr Solzhenitsyn who wrote "as if" an author could examine and publish the history of one's country, and Rosa Parks who sat down on the bus "as if" a diligent black woman could rest after a hard day's work.

"As if" smolders inside us. "As if" radiates confidence; it does not tiptoe around soliciting challenges. "As if" anchors us, keeps center, and wields an attitude.

For the new nurse educator, "as if" seizes root in knowing the self as teacher, learns "as if" there is more fulfillment than exhaustion, and teaches "as if" there is more joy than worry. "As if" does not ask oneself if one is really a nurse educator. By repeatedly broaching this question you may invite knocks and dents from others and grind down your spirit.

How then, can "as if" be cultivated? How can the new nurse educator sustain this core, shore up this internal smoldering confidence, hold on to this anchor with an attitude?

Knowing the self as teacher, being centered in our own "as if," engages several issues that consistently surface for both the emerging and novice educator. By drawing on the perspective of two new nurse educators and incorporating my reflections, this chapter explores the following areas: (1) appeal of the educator role, (2) preparing to teach, (3) getting started, and (4) relationships with teaching colleagues.

I informally interviewed Diane Marcyjanik and Angela Stombaugh when they had just concluded their first year of full-time classroom and clinical teaching in a baccalaureate nursing program. Diane's first year followed immediately after her MSN completion and built on years of community and acute care nursing practice, as well as military service. When Angie finished her first year of full-time teaching, she had established expertise in acute care pediatric nursing, completed her MSN and doctoral coursework, and was well into her dissertation research.

Both Diane and Angie invite us to learn from their experiences, a faculty that Barbara Tuchman presses us to practice. It is with gracious permission that I summarize their comments, and every attempt has been made to present their opinions and experiences thoroughly and accurately. They also reviewed the chapter to help with this effort. Angie and Diane, on behalf of all nurse educators and nursing students everywhere, please accept our gratitude for bestowing your insightful wisdom and divulging your own "as if."

APPEAL OF THE EDUCATOR ROLE

At the outset, many staff nurses disclose that teaching is a distinctive and pleasing aspect of their role. Both Angie and Diane readily remember what initially drew them into education while they were nurses in practice. Angie referred to her ability to "break things down . . . put things in simpler terms . . . direct my teaching to where the learner was" as she oriented nurse interns and supervised nursing students in her role as a staff RN. Diane found that teaching adults was particularly absorbing; as a prenatal education coordinator she liked "knowing" things and sharing that with others.

Going back further, I have my own childhood memories of playing teacher that comically illustrate my affinity for education. Perhaps many of us can recall an amusing personal memory or two. My older sister was an elementary school teacher and, as a 7-year-old, I visited Jennie's classroom on weekends. I remember stretching up on tiptoes at her wooden pedestal podium in front of her classroom lined with 45 (yes, 45!) empty desks. There I chattered my own teacher talk. In that classroom, I scribbled my own chalk talk on her spotless blackboard. In my snoopy audacity, I even lifted the lid on several of those fourth-graders' desks and poked around some science worksheets I found that were graded in my sister's own hand. I imagine that as Jennie turned away and tittered silently, her classroom walls shuddered with fret and laughter.

In addition to the early attraction of teaching, nurse educators also stress the unending rewards of teaching as they move through their career. Both Angie and Diane describe responses and appreciation from students as extremely gratifying. For example, many students acknowledged Angie's positive influence in their lives. Diane related a student's "ah-ha" moment as he linked his microbiology course to the antibiotics he was administering to a patient.

In the same way, we all must remember what tugs us into teaching—what was our "love at first sip"—and recall those satisfiers that continually motivate us, time after time. This recollection plays a part in knowing the self that teaches, carries us on through our "bad days," and directs our own further development.

Besides highlighting their initial teaching abilities, as well as ongoing teaching attractions and rewards, Angie and Diane discussed their own learning as new educators. Angie says, "My own learning stimulates me . . . as I prepare for class I get to find out what's new about the content I'm teaching." Diane concedes, "One of the best things about that first year was learning how to negotiate a clinical site in my home town and working collaboratively with the staff at that site."

Angie and Diane make parallel points. They promptly admit individual teaching skills that they recognized early and continue to practice frequently. And yes, for both of them, students' learning and appreciation satisfy, even flatter. But when Angie and Diane learn and create as teachers, they are inspired even more. They are being teachers, certainly, but also recognizing and designing opportunities to be learners.

Yet, there may be an art in melding who we are as learners with who we are as teachers. Honestly admitting things we don't know is fundamental, of course. Further, being an enthusiastic learner along with the students often facilitates a faculty–student relationship and role models a sense of inquiry.

On the other hand, if we constantly focus solely on our newness, the students tire. If we say again and again, "I've never taught this course or content before," the students fade. And if we constantly respond to students' questions by referring them to their readings because we don't know the answer, they wilt (and often resist).

Instead, reframing who we are as neophytes by capitalizing on our freshness and distinctiveness may edge us closer to the students and secure us closer to the content. For instance, rather than emphasizing our inexperience with acute pain management in children, an alternative response may be, "When I was teaching new RNs on the oncology unit where I worked, we discussed the challenges in managing chronic pain. What I did there to help patients with cancer and their families deal with their pain was. . . . Let's discuss how those strategies that we used on the oncology unit might be similar to or different from managing children's pain right after surgery." By reframing in this way we bring our past expertise to the current learning focus and, at the same time, help students engage and practice making connections.

Confidence in our own reasoning, critical thinking, life experiences, ability to use resources, as well as our own knowing (typically knowing a great deal) must be relished and expressed freely and openly. It is not underscoring *only* who we are as learners (new educators) and it is not underlining *only* our responsibility as teachers—it is etching out the dynamic balance between learner and teacher that keeps us centered, fosters our "as if" stance, further carves out our confidence.

PREPARING TO TEACH

I have been asked frequently about how to prepare for the educator role. As people apply for an academic teaching position or contemplate graduate school, begin coursework, progress further into the program, or delve into teaching in their first year, they often pose the question: "What can I do now that will help me later as a teacher?"

Diane crafted an exemplary MSN program experience to prepare for a teaching position. First, she enrolled in several nursing and nonnursing graduate education courses that provided her the basics (e.g., curriculum development, student evaluation issues, writing test questions, and discovering her own identity as an educator). These courses also helped her know what questions to ask as she began in her teaching position. Second, Diane took advantage of a graduate teaching assistant (TA) position that enabled her to "hang out" with faculty, live in their setting, and study their work. In her TA position, she practiced teaching in the classroom and in a skills lab and studied the students and their questions, priorities, and motivations. Third, Diane served as the student representative on the graduate curriculum committee in which she learned more about curriculum (e.g., program development, evaluation, accreditation), school and university organization, and faculty communication. Finally, Diane was a co-investigator with two other educators and an undergraduate student in a nursing education study. As a researcher, she learned more about the research process, evidence-based teaching, collaboration with faculty and students, and professional presentations and publications. Needless to say, through all of these experiences the faculty in the school learned who she was as a teacher, a leader, a scholar, and a person.

Diane recognizes that she was extremely privileged to have all of these opportunities and that they are not possible for everyone. She adds, however,

"I cannot begin to tell you how worthwhile they were. . . . Through them I learned about myself, education, other faculty, the students, the program, and the wider university." Diane's graduate experience reminds me of the Master-Card advertising campaign, "There are some things money can't buy." Graduate Tuition Fees: $1956; Books: $682; Commuting costs: $516; Childcare expenses: $1406; Learning from extracurricular activities: Priceless.

Unlike Diane, other individuals may not be as closely aligned with the academic setting. However, for nurse practitioners, nurse managers, and staff nurses immersed in practice, there are also numerous opportunities to prepare for the educator role. For example, most nursing programs seek and welcome community members to serve on internal committees. As in Diane's experience, this would reveal not only the content agenda of the committee but also the internal workings of the academic organization as well as an opening to establish a broader professional network. Similar benefits can be gained by providing an occasional lecture on campus; most faculty habitually search for nurse experts in specific areas of practice to serve as guest presenters.

Another opportunity for nurses in practice to prepare for the educator role may be to serve as a clinical preceptor for students or solicit assistance from the nursing program for your clinical project. For example, undergraduate or graduate students can help you conduct a literature review, design a patient education pamphlet, or analyze patient data on your unit. Finally, participating in local professional nursing organizations (e.g., Sigma Theta Tau, the state nurses' association, or specialty organizations) offers collaboration prospects because many of these groups comprise large numbers of nursing faculty. Some of these opportunities may be more difficult if long geographic distances exist between the practice and education setting; others, however, may be possible with conference calls or Web-based connections.

In recommending things to complete *before* pursuing the educator role, Angie laughingly forewarns, "Get married, move, and complete graduate school *first*, if any of these are in your future plans!" Seriously, she suggests taking every advantage of any classroom teaching opportunities. These could be teaching groups in the community, providing workshops or presentations in one's work setting, or presenting at regional, statewide, or national professional conferences. Angie did have two different, short-term clinical teaching appointments before accepting the full-time faculty position, but wished she had an earlier and more in-depth exposure to classroom teaching.

Classroom teaching experience helps the emerging teacher more fully understand the massive preparation time and effort that is required. Well-crafted teaching demands enormous energy. Stimulating students intellectually requires that they read and write a great deal—this necessitates that faculty also read and write a great deal.

As a new faculty, I was told to plan for 3 hours of preparation time for each hour of teaching; in reality, it probably took me 10 to 20 hours to prepare for an hour of class. I'll be the first to admit, a swift learner I am not. After nearly 30 years of teaching, it still takes me nearly that long, although preparing for subsequent teaching of the same content involves more streamlining and more polishing, more grace and elegance—but indispensable preparation nonetheless.

I'd like to interject a brief, albeit vital imperative here about preparing for an academic teaching position. Please clearly understand that teaching is only one responsibility of the educator role. Depending on the employing institution and its philosophy, other responsibilities may include community, university and professional service, as well as academic advising and various aspects of scholarship (i.e., research, publication, and presentation). Clarifying all the dimensions of a potential teaching position well ahead of time is crucial.

An extra word of warning: Unless they are well aware of the faculty role in higher education, most of the students and most of your family and friends will believe that teaching is the sole responsibility of your position. And further, others (including many legislators and the tax-paying public) often will see your "work" limited to the actual times your classes meet (e.g., 9–10 a.m. on Monday, Wednesday, and Friday). They may have little grasp of (or even tolerance for) the vast number of hours you need to prepare for class, plan courses and curriculum, evaluate students' assignments, and keep up-to-date in nursing and teaching practices.

In preparing for the educator role, then, countless opportunities exist both for the student currently enrolled in a graduate program as well as someone who is considering moving from practice to education. These preliminary activities relate to particular aspects of teaching (e.g., classroom teaching, curriculum development, direct work with students) and to broader issues (e.g., faculty collaboration, organizational culture, and personnel issues). Preparing for the educator role requires an intentional seek and search, but this groundwork is priceless. Additionally, a heightened awareness of the demands of teaching is needed. The first year of teaching is a dreadful time to hold several part-time positions or take on a variety of new activities. Finely honed organizational skills and keeping things simple are extremely worthwhile. This is the time to be more realistic than idealistic.

GETTING STARTED: BEFORE THE FIRST CLASS MEETING

Teaching insists on a daily-ness, an absorption. Perhaps this daily raptness with teaching replicates the raptness with painting, or at least as Picasso envisioned painting: "For the true painter, painting is not a gentleman who paints all day long, nor a café get-together, nor an endless babble over 'what is painting?' and 'why do you paint?' To paint or not to paint? To paint this or to paint that? One should paint everything, embrace everything, try everything, lay open the whole earth to our knowledge. . . . When Picasso is not painting, he is painting all the time just the same" (Parmelin, n.d., pp. 86–87). Might it also be thus with teaching—when one is not teaching, he or she is teaching all the time just the same?

This teaching all the time just the same can be grinding, sometimes even crushing, especially for new educators. Angie and Diane disclosed some challenges from their own first year: (1) using someone else's course material and trying to make it "their own," (2) unfamiliarity with the curricular sequence and emphasis, (3) inadequate and inconsistent resource persons, and (4) little acquaintance with the organizational culture and communication patterns. Often new faculty perceive that they fall behind immediately. They admit feeling isolated and marginalized with negligible voice and equate their teaching life to a "triangle being installed into a small square."

To manage these common hurdles in getting started, Angie and Diane recommend several techniques. First, take full advantage of all orientation meetings for new employees, both within the nursing program and campus-wide. Specific agenda items may not directly pertain to you, such as health insurance that you will not be using or library navigation in which you're already skilled. And class preparation may be calling you deafeningly as all your hours of classroom teaching threaten on your to-do list. However, participating in all orientation activities helps establish contacts, build a network, and generate a feeling of belonging—all of which will serve you inestimably in the long term.

Second, ask questions. Because you may have years of nursing practice experience, others frequently assume that you can move into an educator position with little assistance. That is, because you are an expert in practice you will instinctively be an expert in education. From my experience, this seamless and automatic transition is rarely the case. Ask for help, ask specifically, and ask as often as needed.

I've learned that certain ways of posing a question are more successful than other approaches. Framing your question from a *learning perspective* will usually be more acceptable (e.g., "Operating the new teaching station in Room 102 is new to me. Can you please help me learn how to . . ."). *Doing your homework* also helps. Instead of admitting, "I am totally clueless about class rosters," it may be more effective to ask, "I've learned from the university Web site that I need to confirm my class rosters. I tried following their directions but I'm having difficulty tracking the strategy they suggested. Can you please help me with that process?" A strong *student focus* will also strengthen your question.

For example, "I will have several nontraditional students in my class this semester and they may benefit from some of the services provided on campus. I know there is an office in Building X that works with nontraditional students. Can you please tell me what experiences you've had with that service?" Finally, *thinking ahead* avoids last-minute flurry and chaos. Rather than dashing around madly as you search all the file drawers in the department office, it probably will be more effective to plan ahead, for example, "I'm going to be submitting an exam to the test-scoring service in a couple of weeks. Can you tell me please what forms need to be completed with that submission?"

Not only will these approaches result in more patient and useful responses from others, but they also will be highly valued qualities in your own performance review. And, as part of professional courtesy, a follow-up thank-you is indispensable.

New educators sometimes protest (with understandable annoyance and frustration), "Everyone I ask tells me something different!" Policy and procedural operations are always evolving; they are works in progress. It is no different from nursing practice in the healthcare setting where everyone does things a little differently, has developed different shortcuts, and has a different understanding based on personal history, education, and philosophy. In some situations, it may be necessary to ask several people the same question and then form your own conclusion. At other times, just go with the first response.

Another element of asking questions occurs around contentious or thorny issues that surface either openly in meetings or more covertly in hallway conversations. Angie described her effort at always trying to figure out "what's okay to say . . . what's okay to ask . . . where this has been discussed before . . . and whether I am supposed to already know this."

Keeping your eyes open and ears tuned around knotty issues is essential, but also trying to learn more candidly will help you and others. Again, taking a learning perspective, it may work to ask, "This seems to be an important concern and I'd like to learn more about it. Can someone please summarize the history for me and what some of the debates have been?" This approach focuses on the issue and does not emphasize certain individuals. Or, as controversial issues unfold, again it may be useful to ask a question from a student-centered perspective, "Could we discuss what options or solutions might be most meaningful, beneficial, or significant from the student learning standpoint?"

A third technique to address challenges in getting started that the two nurse educators offered was to commit the time and effort to shape your individual classroom teaching style. Angie describes this as "teaching the class as 'your own.'" In describing her getting started experience, Angie raised a concern about receiving course materials from other faculty who previously taught the content, trying to use that material as her primary teaching structure, and then finding the class was not "her own."

I've often heard new educators speak of this predicament. Regrettably, new teachers sometimes wait until the evening before the first class to open someone else's class folder, believing all along that their class preparation was already complete. I don't think you would consider walking into class, opening the textbook for the first time, and trying to teach from it. Perhaps some educators can do this effectively, but, in my own experience and in working with many novice faculty, this has not occurred. In truth, it has often been nearly catastrophic for the teacher and the students. One new faculty confessed, "I was super busy and I thought I could just walk in and teach class from someone else's material. As class began I was quickly circling the drain." I cherish her honesty and empathize with her mortification.

I suggest treating someone else's class folder as simply another resource, comparable to the textbook readings, journal articles, Web site information, and experts in the field. All of these resources provide valuable content information, but information from all the sources must be soaked up and synthesized, organized, and linked with classroom teaching activities to fit your own style. It is these processes that take me 10 to 20 hours to accomplish to prepare for class—yes, when one is not teaching he or she is teaching all the time just the same.

This past semester I had a "here is my course folder" experience. When I took over a course from another faculty, she most charitably gave me the 15-page syllabus and all her course content folders she had used for the 11 years she taught the course. At first, I casually assumed that I would need only to change the dates on the syllabus and it would be ready. After a more thorough review, I instantly realized that her syllabus would not work for me. As Angie labeled it, I needed to make the course, and hence the syllabus, fully "my own."

The course description and objectives remained the same, naturally, but I then began from the bottom up: revising major assignments, moving large online components to a face-to-face format, and changing reading assignments. Overall, I downsized the course significantly. I am teaching the course in this slimmed-down version that I can handle for the first semester. Then, I can develop the course differently after I've had a chance to absorb it. This is another reminder about knowing the self as teacher.

When approaching a course for the first time, "chunking" the course into several topical units also may be helpful. Rather than approaching the course day by day or week by week, divide it into several units with an approximate number of weeks allotted for each unit to make the course more manageable. In this way, you are not carrying the burden of the entire course with you all the time; instead, you can focus on a single unit more deeply and thoroughly and let the other units rest in the margin.

Getting started can be laborious, rocky, even brutal. We know there are few straight lines in teaching—it is filled with swerves and curves, stumbles and staggers. But as the new educator wobbles in and out of the margin, there are explicit strategies that can help in getting started and moving beyond the first year. Plunging into the campus and nursing culture, people, resources, and curricula by developing a network of support is the first step. This, in turn, helps us learn and extend our own teaching style and sustains our "as if" confidence.

RELATIONSHIPS WITH TEACHING COLLEAGUES

Thus far, you have been drawn into education, prepared for the role, and launched the early weeks of your new teaching position. You also have painstakingly and repeatedly introduced yourself to your new teaching colleagues across campus and within the nursing organization. Continual effort is necessary, however, to further establish effective working relationships, or the first year experience may become increasingly detached and forlorn.

Angie and Diane propose several explicit methods to maintain a collaborative approach. First, Angie found that participating in some social activities with others helped her "see beyond their role, learn about their background and their interests." In addition to the occasional house party or connections around specific interests, Angie also noted that attending dinners with candidates interviewing for faculty positions was especially valuable because she learned more about the faculty role in this more casual interview setting while meeting her colleagues in a social milieu.

"Going beyond the silo of nursing," as Diane describes it, is a second strategy that establishes broader collegial relationships. As a graduate student and a first-year educator, she connected with faculty and staff across campus in various ways: participating in university book chats, seeking technical support for courses and professional presentations, attending faculty development seminars and workshops, and enrolling in nonnursing graduate courses. Diane was steadfast in the value of these activities, "For me, it was different people in different disciplines in different buildings that inspired, shared, supported, and collaborated in my education."

All of these established and nurtured relationships provide the footing for leading others and improving teaching and learning. Becoming an educator calls for leadership that is built on relationships and the ability to communicate persuasively.

Diane found herself in situations where she wanted to persuade her colleagues, to sell a specific idea. These situations could be reordering the flow of classroom content to better prepare students for clinical experiences, modifying a written assignment to strengthen critical thinking and prevent plagiarism, or suggesting rewording of some multiple choice test items to enhance clarity and minimize inherent cultural bias.

Going into such discussions fully prepared was key, which required planning rationale and "doing my homework carefully and thoroughly. . . . I needed to know what I was talking about . . . my idea just couldn't be a shapeless shadow."

Convincing others is a persuasive art. A helpful hint to summarize large amounts of information (e.g., rationale, benefits, background, process) is to condense, prioritize, and enumerate two or three key items that the listener or reader can absorb at once. In addition, linking those items with local students, the university strategic plan, a research base, and/or recent concerns raised on campus enhances their appeal. For instance, "There are three major benefits to the students with the approach I'm suggesting. One, which is widely supported by current research, is that . . . The second benefit is particularly suited to the large number of first-generation college students on our campus . . . The third benefit, which has been highlighted in our school evaluation plan, is . . ."

This meticulous and shrewd use of language reminds me of Levitt and Dubner's (2005) discussion about the terminology used by real estate agents. They found a distinct difference between terms correlated with a home's higher sales price (e.g., granite, Corian, maple, state-of-the-art, and gourmet) and those terms correlated with a lower sales price (e.g., fantastic, spacious, charming, great neighborhood, and use of the exclamation point). To persuade most successfully, then, watchfulness about current issues and a wary use of language are indispensable. To sell our idea, we must learn how to portray it as the "granite," the "maple," the "gourmet."

Finally, if your idea is broader in scope with a more significant impact, it may be advantageous to practice your presentation in front of one or two colleagues. They can pose questions and play the devil's advocate before you submit your idea to a larger group.

Being prepared to present your idea verbally in this way is critical. However, if your proposal is complex (e.g., affecting several faculty, courses, and levels of students or requiring phases of implementation), it is also incredibly useful to have a visually friendly one-page handout for distribution. Identified with your name, this handout would contain a brief description of your idea, as well as its background, benefits, research support, resources needed, plan for implementing, and evaluation. The summary provides a written reference for others, connects the idea with you and your name, organizes your verbal comments, and reflects your scholarly diligence.

Establishing effective relationships with teaching colleagues is basic, intricate, and demands purposeful intention. A new faculty (or any faculty, for that matter) wishing to "just simply go into my classroom or clinical with my students and close the door" begs for an instant crash and burn. Engaging in social activities, developing cross-campus connections, and proposing to sell an idea offer a beginning for a successful and meaningful first year.

CONCLUSION

Our "as if," then, is fundamental. It shoulders us as new nurse educators through the first year and beyond. Eva Hoffman (1989), who wrote about her move as a 13-year-old from post–World War II Poland to the American West, describes this centeredness in her memoir. "We all need to find this place in order to know that we exist not only within culture but also outside it. We need to triangulate to something—the past, the future, our own untamed perceptions, another place" (p. 276).

So, as nurse educators we need to pause. We must remember the joys of education as we prepare to teach, get started, and establish relationships with teaching colleagues. That is, we need to discover the bottom of a profession at the same time that we learn it from the top. As we continue to know the self as teacher, we need to triangulate—to simultaneously grip the base and push out the boundaries. We must see how we exist both within the world of education and also off its campus. As we carry on, we will wonder less often what we *should* be like as educators, and it will be "as if" we simply know.

REFERENCES

Hitchens, C. (2001). *Letters to a young contrarian*. New York: Basic Books.

Hoffman, E. (1989). *Lost in translation: A life in a new language*. New York: Penguin Books.

Levitt, S. D., & Dubner, S. J. (2005). *Freakonomics: A rogue economist explores the hidden side of everything*. New York: HarperCollins Publishers.

Moaveni, A. (2005). *Lipstick jihad: A memoir of growing up Iranian in America and American in Iran*. New York: PublicAffairs of the Perseus Books Group.

Parmelin, H. (n. d.). *Picasso: The artist and his model and other recent works*. New York: Harry N. Abrams.

CHAPTER 4

Scott's Spirit on Lassen Peak: Finding the Spirit That Sustains You

It is in fact nothing short of a miracle that the modern methods of instruction have not yet entirely strangled the holy curiosity of inquiry; for this delicate little plant, aside from stimulation, stands mainly in need of freedom; without this it goes to wrack and ruin without fail.

—Albert Einstein

Messages about balancing the different pieces of our life smack us from every direction. Strive for some work, some play, some family, some friends, some exercise, some healthy foods, some sleep, some wine, and on and on. For me, it's less about finding balance—a little of this and a little of that—and more about finding spirit. Knowing the self as teacher, as the focus of Unit 1, propels me to uncover that spirit. This chapter is about discovering what sustains you above all else. I explain my own stumblings about spirit and warmly invite you to stumble and further the search for your own spirit—finding the summit that sustains you.

I've only recently begun to unearth spirit for me. But before I get to that, I'd like to digress and describe how I imagine spirit. I'm borrowing here from David Whyte (1994), who differentiated Strategy from Spirit (he actually termed it Soul) and admonished us to find equal place for both in our lives. According to Whyte, Strategy is age, builds experience, plans its life, gathers knowledge, uses cunning and tactics, waits patiently, and endures hardship for a noble cause. Spirit, on the other hand, is eternally innocent, forever young, vital, inexperienced, foolish, blessed by luck, and often in the right place at the right time. The Spirit doesn't need to keep track of every detail.

As I draw on Whyte's proposals for myself, I envision Strategy as the structure, the tangible, the perseverance, perhaps the labor. It is that little voice advising, "Think carefully now, consider all the details and the consequences."

It is my heart cautioning me to "work hard now, do this now, take the bumps now . . . you will be rewarded in the end." For me, Strategy assembles networks, grinds through graduate degrees, and tramps down a tenure track. Strategy is critical, but it must be blended with Spirit. Yet, I continually search, what is Spirit? And I probe further, what is Spirit for me?

LESSON FROM LASSEN PEAK

A preschooler taught me about Spirit many years ago on Lassen Peak. Lassen stretches up more than 10,000 feet in a northern California national park, and, in some shady spots, snow stays safe year-round there. Looming 1000 feet above its surroundings, the peak makes a bold statement. Its volcanic energy both created and destroyed the land in its fiery past.

My sister Jennie, her three young children, my husband, Wayne, and I visited the peak on a scorching August day in 1979. The "Climb a Volcano" announcement in the park brochure snared us with cleverly tempting trail bait: well-graded path, only 2.5 miles, "see the top in less than two hours," suitable for all ages. Being natives of Wisconsin, where the tallest peak is Timm's Hill at 1952 feet, we were eager, albeit greenhorn mountain hikers. We disregarded the wisdom of wearing sturdy shoes, bringing water and food, and most other requirements of a 2000-foot climb that first *began* at 8500 feet elevation. Dim-witted, we set off.

Up and down, the peak climb was brutal. For the first few switchbacks, the kids in their excitement impatiently dashed to the next bend in the trail and then ran back to meet us. It wasn't long though, perhaps only another 50 yards, until they asked a descending couple, "Are we almost to the top?" Dressed in name-brand hiking shorts and up-scale hiking boots and drinking from designer water bottles, the couple gently smiled their encouragement, "No, you have a ways to go, but you'll make it." We should have interpreted that cheer differently, but parched, cramped, and blistered, we trudged foolishly forward in the searing high noon sun. Bump, bump, bump, we flip-flopped up and up the stony path.

The kids quickly slowed to a slog. In fact, Wayne, Jennie, and I took turns carrying Scott, the youngest at $3\frac{1}{2}$ years old—he just couldn't walk another step. He actually napped on our shoulders as we jolted upward, stone by stone. Scott didn't even open his eyes when we swapped him among us at every switchback and then paused to shake out our own throbbing arms and stamp our aching legs in relief.

Six hours later, we landed back at the bottom, full of stunning sights and a celebrated sense of accomplishment, but all of us were dangerously drained and depleted. As we clomped back to our car in the now nearly empty parking lot Wayne teased, with a wink and a withering dehydrated smile, "I left my car keys at the top of the peak. I need to go back up to get them." Scott, the little one we carried most of the way to the top and back down again, looked up with his bed-head hair and sparkling eyes in a flushed dry face. He enthusiastically volunteered, "I'll go back and get the keys for you, Uncle Wayne."

That is Spirit. That is the eternal innocence and youthful foolishness jumping to go back up and retrieve the car keys from the top of Lassen Peak. Although our volcano climb was stony-slim on Strategy, Scott showed me Spirit—the need to make my own way in the world and be alert to my own future, no matter what the obstacles. Whyte (1994) asserts that it is this Spirit, forever young, that outlives the life that is held down by experience, a life often hindered by Strategy.

Sometimes with the spotlight on Strategy, there are the most miserable tragedies. For those of us who have been driven solely by Strategy and who have neglected Spirit throughout our careers, there is no one left inside to cherish the treasures when we can finally relish our lives. Or, if we long neglected our Spirit or our employing organization strangled it day by day or year by year, we come to a time when the Strategy in our life is no longer needed in the same way, and we assume our life is over.

At the end of the day, then, we must bring our innocence and experience together—knitting our Spirit and our Strategy into a whole—in all facets of our life, not just when we are not at work. If we uncover and sustain the Spirit only outside of work, perhaps when we snatch a vacation or steal a 3-day weekend, then we deny ourselves fulfillment in the place where we spend most of our time and energy. This denial produces a dehydrated work life.

LEARNING AS MY SUSTAINING SPIRIT

I'm just beginning to uncover Spirit, and for me Spirit is learning. Learning is the vitality, the questioning, the youthful innocence in my life. Learning seasons the Strategy, flavors the structure, and spices up my methodical planning.

This Spirit is not only about *me* learning, but it's also about *others* learning. It's not only learning in the workplace, but it's learning everywhere. It's not only the new content that I'm learning, but it is how I'm learning. The excitement around the process of learning spreads between and among the students and me. Yes, I can weave in content or the "what" I've learned, say, inject a bit about Middle Eastern culture into a research unit that I'm teaching, but it is in teaching "how" and "why" I'm learning that enlivens the classroom for the students and for me.

So, how and why *am* I learning? What is this Spirit of learning for me? During a recent semester, I along with my sister Jennie, who recently retired as an elementary school teacher, audited a history class on my campus. The youthfulness of auditing a history class with undergraduate students was Spirit for me. Also Spirit was the relative inexperience of registering for the course, finding the books, and learning about knowledge generation in the discipline of history (i.e., how do historians come to know?). And of course, as an auditor, I didn't need to keep track of every detail as a Strategist would be called to do.

So, every Tuesday evening for 15 weeks Jennie drove 200 miles from the southern part of the state and we trudged off to class together, with our old-school tote bags in hand and a haughty spring in our step. The department chair, Dr. Katherine (Kate) Lang, taught History 385, History of Middle Eastern Muslim Women. Actually, all the 30-plus undergraduate students in the class were also my "teachers" (many were history majors and juniors or seniors). The students taught me how imperative it is to (1) repeat confusing or complex points even when I become impatient with multiple requests to do so (e.g., differences in the origins of major world religions or the timeline of key events in Islam), (2) prepare students for exams by highlighting content and providing study questions, and (3) honor their ability to simplify and design new models of making connections (and yet I must be careful to attend to accuracy, bias, and stereotypes in their simplification).

Auditing the history class propelled me to examine my own learning, but it also directed me to reflect on students' learning.

WHAT I HAVE LEARNED ABOUT LEARNING

I'd like to offer a few ideas I've learned about learning and how it is becoming my Spirit. First, learning something I don't know delights me and stimulates me further—this is the vitality of Spirit. For example, previously to me *Sunni* and *Shiite* meant little more than groups of people who lived somewhere in the Middle East. Now I know that Sunnism and Shiism both enforce and interpret law, but that shii law leaves more room for interpretation and sunni law is more bound by tradition. Early leadership of the two groups is grounded in different people and beliefs, and different practices exist around homes, cars, mosques, and prayer. Because of the history class, every time I hear or read the terms *Sunni* or *Shiite* I briefly review what the terms mean (and I feel proud to be able to do that), and so the learning continues through reinforcement. Before the class, I ignored these two terms, "tuning them out," because I didn't know the difference between them or what they meant.

Learning with Kate, Jennie, and all the students in the class has kindled me further. Since the history class, Jennie and I have a long-distance weekly phone chat as we move through the chapters of Sandy Tolan's *The Lemon Tree* (2006), a historical, nonfiction narrative of Arabs and Jews in the heart of the Middle East. We understand the book more now because of the history class we audited together, and this fact convinces me once again about learning as Spirit. This learning makes me feel more and sense more and to be more a part of the world.

I must admit I used to sneer when the nursing students told me that everything stopped for them on Thursday evenings when they could watch the television show *ER* or whatever the latest health-related show happened to be. How could they be so glued to this scrap of "Hollywood health care"?

When I finally could hear beyond my sneer, I learned that the students would review the medical and nursing content and terms they saw and heard while watching the show (usually with each other). For example, were the dosages of drugs accurate? Was the route of administration appropriate? Did the pathophysiology and symptoms of the diseases in the characters make sense based on what they knew? Of course, the students elatedly predicted much of the action and triumphed when they noticed an error. I am convinced they could all have been expert consultants to the show.

Now I get it. The students were reviewing new content through reinforcement. This invigorated them, just as I am also elated when I understand more clearly the Sunni or Shiite highlighted on the evening news or appreciate more deeply the Arab Muslim and Jewish experience in a book I'm reading. I will sneer no more.

Second, learning also gives me confidence, a sense of self-assurance to speak up. Perhaps this is honoring the inexperienced part of my spirit. Throughout most of my life, I have been hesitant to voice my opinion or contribute verbally in a group discussion. One of my faculty in a long-ago graduate nursing theory course, Dr. Merle Mishel at California State University–Los Angeles, counseled me about this in a most gracious and affirming way: "You have so much to offer." (Although I was ecstatic to hear this, I really didn't believe her—was this doubt part of my first-generation college student syndrome?) She advised me further, "Plan to ask a question early in our class discussion, and then you can rest easier. Questions are just as valuable as other comments." Her guidance occurred nearly 30 years ago. I'm reminded once again that teaching lasts an eternity. Thank you, Merle, for helping me examine my own confidence and participation and practice some strategies despite a racing pulse rate that, to this day, sometimes rams me into a tachy panic.

Now I more readily notice self-belief and assurance considerations in students and try to discuss them openly and honestly. I begin with describing for the student what I'm observing. Trying not to be preachy, I affirm the need for students to find their voice and highlight some approaches that they can practice (e.g., asking questions as suggested by Dr. Mishel, sharing an experience with the class from their own practice with patients). Inevitably, my own struggles with confidence creep into my discussion with students and help confirm our humanity.

I recall two additional examples about learning and confidence, both related to the history class I was taking. I am a member of our largely male University Planning Committee, and at a recent meeting the need to increase student diversity on our campus, with a focus on black and Hispanic students, was being discussed. (Diversity has probably been on more university agendas around the nation than any other item, except perhaps budget.) With a hammering heart, I added that we must also consider Middle Eastern culture and East African students because there are growing numbers of Somalian immigrants in our geographic area. I sensed a thoughtful pause of agreement and my confidence inched up a notch. So far, so good.

In the second example, I was teaching about culture diversity and leadership in a graduate class and discussed how differences in dress and appearance may influence leadership. I described someone wearing a *hijab* and the meanings it may hold for Muslim women. Before my history class I was uncertain about the term *hijab* and would never have felt comfortable using this illustration. In both examples, learning has pressed my confidence forward and at the same time respected the inexperience of my spirit.

Third, learning has an innocent twist to it—it makes my spirit smile. In the Middle Eastern history class, regularly humbled by my own lightweight knowledge level, I repeatedly marveled at the other students' in-depth understanding. A couple times I have also smiled at their learning (and recalled my own unmistakable innocence in similar situations). For example, in discussing harems and all their attendants, one young woman was unclear about the definition of *eunuch* and asked in our class discussion, "Is a eunuch like a little army?" She was a tad embarrassed to learn about the boys whose testicles were removed, but she had the eunuchs' guarding army role in the harem right on. I suspect this young woman was not the only student in the class that gasped slightly at this revelation.

But it was this same young woman who quietly demurred in a class discussion the following week: "You can always tell a great deal about a people by the way they treat their most vulnerable individuals or groups." Innocence of spirit, yes, but eloquent wisdom, too.

Fourth, learning helps me see the flipside, the reverse, how it feels to sit in the student's seat. As a teacher, I savored being a student in the history class. Not only was I co-learning about the history of Middle Eastern Muslim women with my sister, but I was also seeing Dr. Katherine Lang, a master teacher at work. As a student, I was learning about teaching.

What did I learn about teaching? Although it was a history class, the content was not taught chronologically. We read four books for the class, interspersed with essays authored by Middle Eastern women. This approach invited me to think more openly about content organization and moving beyond the organizational approaches with which I am most familiar: individual to family, or cell to organ systems, or simple to complex.

I'd like to momentarily digress here on the topic of the traditional "simple to complex" continuum. In his recent book *Simplexity: Why Simple Things Become Complex (and How Complex Things Can Be Made Simple)*, Jeffrey Kluger (2008) exposes the paradox and blunders in how we've typically regarded simplicity and complexity. For example, because we venerate size and speed and scale, we see a star as more complex than a guppy despite the guppy's myriad biological systems and subsystems. Yet, it is likely that the guppy is far more complex. Similarly, a houseplant with its detailed metabolism and chemical processes may be far more complex than a manufacturing plant.

Simplexity, then, redefines how we look at the world and provokes us to review our notions of simple to complex in nursing curricula. Are activities of daily living (ADL) skills really more simple than helping a client manage a chronic illness? Or is history taking more simple than learning intensive care monitoring? And, perhaps even more significantly, is a simple-to-complex curricular organization meaningful—is this organization itself simple or complex?

In the history class, I also learned about the teacher's sway in upholding students. Kate affirmed students in many different ways, such as learning and using students' names and inviting (no, expecting) questions. She responded to all questions fully and respectfully, beginning with "That's a great and very important question." No question was ever branded as stupid, with a "you should already know this." In her encouraging style, Kate frequently and rock-solidly stated, "You can do this. You know this. You can write scholarly responses to the essay question based on your readings and class discussions." As a student in the class, I never wavered or dithered in who I was, what I knew, and where I needed to go in my learning.

I learned another lesson about teaching while sitting in the student's seat. As a co-student with my sister in the class, I noticed that it was well into the second half of the semester before Jennie made a verbal comment out loud in class. Often, she would mouth her comment or whisper her response to me only, but would not say it audibly to the entire class. How many other students also respond in a similar way? As teachers, we might think the students are being rude, whispering to each other about unrelated content, not paying attention, or talking about last night's date. But perhaps they actually lack self-confidence. Perhaps these students indeed are fully engaged in the class content, thinking and even talking with each other about it. It may be wiser to invite them in and create safe opportunities for participation rather than to hush or silence them.

Fifth and finally, learning wakes up the foolishness, the flippant, the windfall, the luck of Spirit for me. It helps to be in the right place at the right time. Throughout my elementary and high school years, I played a flute in a small, rural school with a far-south-of-middling band program. I barely learned the basics, repeating those bare and boring basics for 8 years. After my high school graduation, the flute laid fallow for nearly 30 years as its pads dried and my mouth formation and breathing technique became ancient history. Then, I was invited to play three songs at a wedding. Yikes! My dear musician friend Lee Anna's intense and tender drilling helped me fumble through the flute fingerings at the ceremony. It was far from a polished performance, but at least was not a dreadful embarrassment to the bride, groom, or me.

That nuptial bumbling piqued my relearning, and with Lee Anna's prodding, I landed in a community concert band. I won't budge from the last chair position, even as new members join the flute section. Bonded to that chair, I could sneak by with playing only some of the notes, don't need to keep track of every detail, and know the rest of the band will carry on, resulting in a striking rendition of Verdi or Handel. Propped by luck and feeling a trifle foolish, my spirit of learning deemed I was in the right place at the right time.

Learning then, in all of its intricacy, is the Spirit that sustains me. Learning carries me to a place where I am a stranger and there delights and stimulates me to explore and to find out. Learning gives me confidence in my inexperience. It plays with my innocence, reverses my spin, and stirs up my luck and foolishness. It helps me see that the time and place may be right and that I can let go of some of the details.

Learning escorts me to the classroom year after year so that I can teach and learn with the students; it will outlive my Strategy life that structures, organizes, maneuvers, and manipulates, although that too is essential for me. Learning, honoring Einstein's "holy curiosity of inquiry," makes me want to follow Scott up Lassen Peak to retrieve the car keys again and again.

In *Truck: A Love Story*, author Michael Perry (2006; p. 239) got right to the heart of learning as sustaining Spirit when he portrayed a group he hung out with over the years at the corner table at The Joynt. "They had remained engaged . . . whether they earned their buck from behind a lectern or on a scaffold, they hadn't allowed their brains to kick into neutral. They hadn't become satisfied . . . this was not on the whole a churchly crew, but they had a fundamental understanding of sin, the greatest of which was to play dumb."

FIND THE SPIRIT THAT SUSTAINS YOU

From his deathbed Morrie Schwartz (Albom, 1997) candidly championed a message similar to Perry's (2006). In this biographical novel, Morrie was the aging and dying sociologist professor whom the writer Mitch Albom visited over several weeks. In this dying and deathbed vigilance Mitch, a former student of Morrie's, learned some of the richest lessons of life.

In one of their Tuesday discussions, with Morrie curled on his side, small and withered in more of a boy's body than a man's, Mitch sadly reminisced about his own work life, "Over the years, I had taken labor as my companion and had moved everything else to the side" (p. 43). Perhaps Mitch was awakening to the misery of a strangled Spirit and a Strategy that shrouded his life.

With short breaths that stabbed each raspy phrase, Morrie responded, "You have to be strong enough to say if the culture doesn't work, don't buy it. . . . devote yourself to creating something that gives you purpose and meaning . . . so many people walk around with a meaningless life. They seem half-asleep, even when they're busy doing things they think are important. This is because they're chasing the wrong things" (pp. 42, 43).

Discovering Spirit for yourself begins with knowing the self. To what extent have we become simply satisfied with Strategy and have little Spirit to sustain us? Are we sleepwalking through our busy Strategy, or do we have the Spirit to turn around, once again, to follow Scott back up to Lassen Peak? When I hear middle-aged (or any age, for that matter) individuals lament the many years before they can retire, I can't help but question their lack of Spirit or dominance of Strategy. In no way do I mean to minimize the goodness of retirement, but might we be spending all our life simply "waiting to retire . . . I can't wait till that time comes . . . standing at the gate till it opens?"

Perhaps asking ourselves some of the age-old questions is a place to begin. What makes us most happy (and then augmenting that while curtailing the other)? What draws other people closer to us? What do we want our grandchildren to remember about us? Finding that individual sustaining Spirit calls us to stumble and stop, and then study our chase.

REFERENCES

Albom, M. (1997). *Tuesdays with Morrie: An old man, a young man, and life's greatest lesson.* New York: Doubleday.

Kluger, J. (2008). *Simplexity: Why simple things become complex (and how complex things can be made simple).* New York: Hyperion.

Perry, M. (2006). *Truck: A love story.* New York: Harper Perennial.

Tolan, S. (2006). *The lemon tree: An Arab, a Jew, and the heart of the Middle East.* New York: Bloomsbury.

Whyte, D. (1994). *The heart aroused: Poetry and the preservation of the soul in corporate America.* New York: Doubleday.

CHAPTER 5

The Rhythm of Education: Dr. Harriet Werley, Thank You for Teaching Me

Setting an example is not the main means of influencing another, it is the only means.

—Albert Einstein

In pausing to reflect on the self as teacher, I bow to others who have molded who I am. A generous mentor and a wise teacher, Dr. Harriet Werley is one of several people who has further "hurt me" into nursing education. In this chapter, I describe what Dr. Werley did, how she did it, and how I've changed as a result. That description further channels ideas for the novice nurse faculty.

I met Dr. Werley in my work as a research assistant with her at the University of Wisconsin–Milwaukee when I was a doctoral student in the late 1980s. Since that time, I've cherished her as one of the elders in my life who continually shapes who I am as an educator. If she were living today and I asked about her mentoring and teaching gifts, I suspect that she would smile unassumingly and say, "I don't understand your question. I'm not doing anything special, it is simply daily-ness that happens in an ordinary way." Dr. Werley, I honor you here with a tribute to that daily-ness.

As this tribute unfolds, you are invited to study those who have been your teachers and mentors, who too might say their daily-ness happens in ordinary ways. Our study, our "ability to revere" as Sarah Vowell (2002, p. 21) terms it, honors those who teach us, how they teach, and how we learn. As a result, our reflective pause intensifies and we learn still more about our self as teacher and about those who learn with us.

THANK YOU FOR TEACHING ME

"Thank you for teaching me." A loving story echoes these words.

47

I visited Dr. Werley a couple years before she died. I will respectfully call her Harriet because that is what she wanted. At that time, Harriet lived in a nursing home and suffered significant cognitive and physical losses. She did not know who I was or where she was or what day or season it was. As Harriet lay curled in her bed after eating two meager spoonfuls of lunch, I sat at her side, and I foolishly regressed to outdated orientation approaches that were used in the past with people who were confused. I dimly and systematically reoriented her by explaining who I was, where we were, and what season it was. I can't believe I stumbled into that archaic and ineffective mode of communication, but I did.

Despite my antiquated reorientation maneuvers, Harriet kindheartedly recognized my efforts. She tilted up on one brittle bony elbow, looked at me brightly, eye to eye, and whispered hoarsely, "Thank you for teaching me."

I gulped back stinging tears and sighed softly, "Harriet, you are *my* teacher, you have taught *me* over all these years. Harriet, thank *you* for teaching *me*."

And then her eyes faded and her face sunk as she silently turned away. I stood, lightly kissed her forehead, and tiptoed away with a sorrowing heart and an anguished spirit. I knew I would never see Harriet again.

But her "teaching me" lives on. Rhythm serves as a fitting metaphor for that teaching because Harriet and her principles command permanence, forte, cadence, and pattern. It is in the Rhythm of Staccato, the Rhythm of Tapestry, and the Rhythm of Stillness that Harriet created daily-ness in ordinary ways. In these rhythms, Harriet's "teaching me" lives on; as Einstein asserted, perhaps her example has been one of the only means that influenced me.

RHYTHM OF STACCATO

The Rhythm of Staccato illustrates Harriet's striking, detached, no-nonsense directives. This rhythm incited me to teach with definition and purpose. It also taught me to be rigorous and detailed, careful and clear, resourceful and incisive.

At the stroke of 8 o'clock every morning, Harriet stepped off the elevator, filled her stained cup from the students' crusty coffee pot, and marched into the tiny windowless office I shared with two other research assistants. Her tattered 1983 edition of the *Publication Manual for the American Psychological Association* formed to her hands. Dozens of hand-torn, odd-shaped little paper markers peeked from all sides of her manual, each distinguished by a penciled word or two. Not one single flashy Post-it note there. I believe she remembered every rule contained therein; as a matter of fact, she probably wrote some of those rules while she served on the APA Manual Board.

I ardently recall Harriet's notes to me, crammed with detailed comments and arrows, written the night before on the back of grocery store receipts. When I heard that elevator bell chime and the door swish open, I twitched up a little straighter and tweaked up a little sharper.

Using those grocery store notes and her APA manual, which always seemed to fall open to the exact page she needed, Harriet would review with me the latest manuscript she was writing for publication, word by word and line by line. She not only related the rule to me from memory, but she described the "why," its history, other illustrating examples, and the page number in the manual where the rule was delineated. Even when my impatience occasionally gnawed and chomped in silence, Harriet taught me to learn the rules and be painstakingly meticulous.

As I learned the rules from Harriet, I also emphasize some of the basic writing guidelines and the APA manual rules with students that I teach. Almost without an exception, I use scholarly papers as a learning activity in both undergraduate and graduate classes. I spend some class time highlighting the principal rules, making available sample papers in hard copy and online, and building on lessons learned in English composition courses. Spending this class time not only helps to describe the detail of the style but also indicates the importance for the students. To the students' common annoyance with some of the writing format details, I respond unswervingly but with empathy for their own gnawing and chomping, "In some things in nursing there is a great deal of leeway, but in other areas—like medication administration—details are critical. So it is with writing. We have flexibility, but we also must vigilantly attend to some particulars and fine points." The students get it and we move on.

Harriet included me as a co-author for several of her publications. Until then I was not published. I will always remember her celebration the first time my name appeared in print in the professional literature. She spryly marched off the 8 o'clock elevator, brandishing "our" article in hand.

To this day my teaching includes helping students move their writing and scholarly pursuits forward in the publication process. Our faculty role in higher education encompasses service and scholarship and offers many teaching opportunities. This teaching may begin by helping students revise a solid paper they have written as a course assignment or inviting a student with a shared interest to participate in ongoing research, paper presentations, or writing. As new educators launch their own scholarly and service careers, the students can become apprentices or partners—often co-learning as the work expands.

For example, after completing my doctorate I presented several professional papers nationally and a report of my gerontological dissertation research was in press. However, there was still an opportunity in this research to further analyze a subset of my data (i.e., focusing on only the women in the study). I connected with a nontraditional undergraduate student interested in women's health, research, and gerontology. Together we analyzed the data subset, presented a professional paper regionally, and co-authored an article in the professional literature.

Harriet's lessons about being careful and clear in this co-scholarship process continue to teach me. It is critical to plan upfront for an effective teacher–student partnership surrounding writing and research. I strive to link with a student(s) that is curious about my content, is attracted to the demands of scholarship, and has demonstrated some "stick-to-itiveness." Marking out a structured timeline together holds us both to steady progress and superior quality work. The times I took a more carefree, happy-go-lucky approach the semester floated by with only a mad flurry of paltry activity in the final week or two. Even with the best of plans and intentions in the sturdiest of partnerships, we have not always been successful (but I have always learned something). Finally, a stern word of caution: In co-authoring with students, everyone's time and detailed effort must be arranged in advance and distributed equitably or the risk for misusing and taking advantage of students is too great. Unfortunately, I have witnessed this exploitation far too many times.

In her Rhythm of Staccato, Harriet also reminded me to be prudent and sparing (e.g., recall the grocery store receipts, as well as ever-lasting polyester clothes and lunch bags reused to the point that they were just bits and crumbs). I relished her frugality—actually, I was charmed by it because her thriftiness bolstered many of my own childhood lessons. In my family, saving rainwater for our baths was a given. My father walked the roads picking up aluminum cans, collected wooden chips at the local ski factory for our kitchen wood-stove, and stockpiled spoiled canned vegetables from the nearby cannery where he worked to feed our farm animals (their stomachs of steel always astounded me as the animals gulped each scrumptious bite). I will spare you the sights, sounds, and smells as my brother, father, and I opened those cans in our cellar.

Now I use these "lessons learned in my family kindergarten" to see the deeply layered meaning of Jean-François Millet's *The Gleaners*. In this mid-19th-century oil painting, the artist gives voice to the impoverished by painting three stooped women gathering what is left of the harvest grains, gleaning anything that was useful. Using light and pivotal placement of the women, Millet portrays the rigors of the poor and working class center stage; up to this time the servants were depicted only as subservient to the royalty or upper class.

As it happened, Harriet and my parents were gleaners of the 20th century, practicing resourceful green-ness long before it was in vogue, years before the term "freegan" was fashioned, and decades before carbon footprints and global warming graced nearly every issue of *Time* magazine. Now green practices come naturally to me and they affirm my family values that once were a painful and disgraceful source of embarrassment with my childhood and teen peers. At that time I tried to be invisible, to fade and blend with others. In this Rhythm of Staccato, Harriet helped me feel normalized. I chuckle now about the quirkiness and peculiarity of things coming full circle.

Consequently, I've learned to appreciate the extent to which students also have been shaped by their culture, their family kindergartens. I fully realize the students do not "check" their families, their culture, and their identity at the door as they enter my classroom. The students come as wholes, and obviously I do not wish for it any other way.

Nobel-laureate Nadine Gordimer (2005) captures this fact when she describes the language of Thapelo, one of her characters in *Get a Life*: "These words in the slang of his mother tongues (he speaks at least four or five) aren't italicized in Thapelo's talk, they belong in English just as his natural use of the scientific terms and jargon of his profession does. Or maybe they're part of the identification with his boyhood street life of blacks he asserts as essential to who and what he is. It's not what he's emancipated from: it's what he hasn't, won't leave behind" (p. 83).

When students begin an assignment I frequently ask them to relate something about their family and culture—what they haven't or won't leave behind—to significant aspects of their learning. This relating is a key component of liberal education. Students often feel safer exploring their connections with family, culture, and identity more exhaustively in their writing rather than verbally. For example, students could be asked to compare parenting practices described in selected research to those in their own family as well as a client family in their public health nursing practice. As they explore, students could also predict their own or others' parenting abilities or appraise their current skills as a parent.

The Rhythm of Staccato is reflected in a poem by William Stafford (1998, p. 42) titled "The Way It Is."

> *There's a thread you follow. It goes among*
> *things that change. But it doesn't change.*
> *People wonder about what you are pursuing.*
> *You have to explain about the thread.*
> *But it is hard for others to see.*
> *While you hold it you can't get lost.*
> *Tragedies happen; people get hurt*
> *or die; and you suffer and get old.*
> *Nothing you do can stop time's unfolding.*
> *You don't ever let go of the thread.*

The thread in Stafford's poem embodies Harriet's Rhythm of Staccato. It's her style, if you will, a creation from within. Fashion changes, style remains. Fashion is imposed from without and demands unthinking subordination. Style springs from self-awareness and individual expression.

This style, this thread, this staccato that is Harriet's daily-ness is our definition and purpose, our rigor and detail, our clarity and urgency, even when others may not see it. If we are never to let go of the thread, as Stafford proposes, we must continuously pause, reflect, and refine the self that teaches.

RHYTHM OF TAPESTRY

Harriet's Rhythm of Tapestry taught me to relate, to interlace, to teach with synthesis and integration. Harriet helped me fit things together, to bond the "and's" in my life: nursing practice *and* research, reading *and* writing, providing answers *and* asking questions, the past *and* the future, inside the classroom *and* outside the classroom. In her scholarship, for example, she merged the details of research and writing with the big picture of nursing and health care. As I look back I envision Harriet's life as a blend of everything and marvel at her centeredness in that blend. Never seeming apologetic, she was who she was.

The epitome of the tapestry lesson I learned from Harriet fuses who I am as teacher, who I am as nurse, and who I am as person. A recent personal experience (with nurses' names changed) anchors that fusion.

After being hospitalized for one final time last July, my father-in-law was being discharged with home hospice services back to our home where he lived with us. Orval was at peace with his dying and death and wished for nothing more than just to get home, after 2 hospital weeks of futile needle poking and pill pushing.

Now more intimately than ever, I was the daughter-in-law and the nurse in the family. After receiving all of the hospice information and agreeing to this service, Orval and I met with the intake RN in his hospital room. It appeared to be her responsibility to describe the final details of hospice care—the "who, when, and where" as we prepared for discharge the following day. Listening to her description, Orval quietly gasped each breath as his swollen, leaden legs flattened the sagging pillows at the foot of his bed. I felt his enduring trust in me, abiding love for his son Wayne (my husband), and gratitude for our home and flower gardens that awaited him after discharge.

After briefly introducing herself as Lori, the intake RN told us that there would be one RN (Jill) seeing Orval at our home the next day to admit him to the hospice service. Then, the following day a second RN (Tina) would be our nurse case manager, would visit our home, and would be our primary nurse.

As a daughter-in-law and as a nurse, I searched for more detail, more identity, and more fullness in our hospice nursing care. I asked Lori for Jill's and Tina's last names. After a heavy and revolting pause, Lori looked directly at me and retorted, "Is that important?" I was instantly muted, but I wanted to screech, "Yes, yes, yes . . . it's very important!" In that split second, I shriveled to a child whose hand had been whacked in public—shamed, diminished, disrespected, and angry. As the child, I could feel my throat squeeze and my eyes brim with tears. I had been silenced by a colleague in the most piercing way possible. Lori proceeded with describing the planning details but never did provide the two RNs' last names. I heard little more of her discussion and couldn't wait for her to leave the room.

My head told me that Jill and Tina were professional nurses and that Orval and I had every right to know their professional identity, including their last names. How could I call the hospice office and ask to speak with "Jill" or "Tina," as if they were table servers in a restaurant? Even more intensely, my heart told me that they would be guests in our home, nurse professionals helping us with Orval's dying and death, arriving during one of the most aching and agonizing times for all of us. And we would not or could not know their last names? They knew our last names. We know the last name of our Culligan water softener technician, our car repairman, our newspaper delivery person. Wasn't my request for the nurses' last names reasonable? How could this be?

With my question for last names, I pleaded to know the nurses' solid professional identities and for a more complete collaboration. Those nurses were to help Wayne and me care for Orval as he died in our own bedroom in our own home. Yes, this information was profoundly important for me as a person and a nurse.

Now as I review Harriet's Rhythm of Tapestry, who I am as person, as nurse, and as teacher mingles and merges. Numerous opportunities exist to entwine this "nurses' last name" experience with my teaching. Harriet would help me pose several challenges that could be explored with students in writing, class discussion, or small group activities. How was I as the client nurse affected over the next several days? How is nurse professional identity established and how is it violated? How does being silenced surface as a concept in the nurse–client relationship? How do nurses understand what the client needs to know? How do clients who are nurses cope with suboptimal health care?

Of course, students also come with their own experiences as part of their personal-professional Tapestry. We must help the students delve into these experiences so that they too can see the "and's" in their own life, move toward a place where their outside matches who they are on the inside, and be more clear about the thread they are gripping.

RHYTHM OF STILLNESS

Finally, Harriet's Rhythm of Stillness taught me to be life giving, to affirm. Silence and solitude are part of this rhythm because they help us to open inner guidance and replenish our spirit and self.

In my silence and stillness, I am learning that there is contentment and peace in detachment, acceptance, letting go. This is not a detachment that is uncaring or callous. It is a detachment from a rigidly designed outcome; it is one that dismantles some certainty.

I am learning to detach from the good old days. Sometimes we profess those days as bright, flawless, crisp-as-an-apple wonderful when, in truth, they were also blurred, murky, and tilted. With this detachment, I am learning about the self as teacher, my style, and the thread I must never let go, but at the same time, I know that the intelligence and courage and perseverance of future nurses and teachers will carry on. I am slowly learning to care deeply from a detached place.

I would like to end now with a loving affirmation I received from Harriet. I had just completed my comprehensive exams after my doctoral coursework at UW-Milwaukee and was launching dissertation research. Together we were walking out to my car in the parking lot by the nursing building one warm day in late May 1988. Harriet stopped at her car first and pulled out a most beautiful brown leather briefcase that she gave to me that I treasure to this day. Inside the briefcase was a card.

In 1988, the briefcase and the card were a gift to me. But now I give Harriet's Rhythm of Stillness to all of you and to all the students she affirmed over the years. On the front of the card, under a beautiful red rose, it said, "You made it!" Inside the card, it said, "I knew you would!"

In her own handwriting was the following message: "As a very talented individual you can do and be anything you want to be; keep up the good work. It has been my pleasure to have had you work with me as a Research Assistant. And, you have contributed so much through it. Best wishes to you as you continue your work on the dissertation and thereafter function in your faculty role. I will watch for your contributions to the profession and the healthcare field. Harriet W."

Harriet, thank you for teaching me. In your Rhythm of Staccato, you have helped me learn about purpose, rigor, detail, and carefulness. In your Rhythm of Tapestry, you have taught me about the "and" in relationships, how to fit things together, how to blend and merge who I am. And in your Rhythm of Stillness, you have helped me examine my self and you have helped me to let go.

Harriet, your absence has become a constant presence. You've bestowed an elegant and inspiring legacy, and I will work to keep that legacy alive. As the card said, you knew I would. You believed in me. And that is the Rhythm of Education.

REFERENCES

Gordimer, N. (2005). *Get a life*. London: Bloomsbury Publishing.

Stafford, W. (1998). *The way it is: New and selected poems by William Stafford*. St. Paul, MN: Graywolf Press.

Vowell, S. (2002). *The partly cloudy patriot*. New York: Simon & Schuster.

Relationships with Students

CHAPTER 6

How Can the Students Help Us Teach?

Instruction begins when you, the teacher, learn from the learner; put yourself in his place so that you may understand . . . what he learns and the way he understands it.

—Søren Kierkegaard

When we publish and speak with each other as nurse educators, we frequently emphasize the teacher perspective. In those publications and dialogues, we communicate with another teacher—often about students. Yet time and again, we overlook the students' view. Or if we do present their angle, and it happens to be critical or unfavorable, we may minimize it, chip it off, or even white-wash it, as if teacher knows best. My goal here is to balance the faculty perspective by giving broad and open voice to the students—as Kierkegaard, the 19th-century Danish philosopher and humanist proclaimed—to learn from the learners, to understand the way they understand.

I recently interviewed two seniors who were graduating from our baccalaureate nursing program, were students in my class, and whom I knew for 3 years: Krystle Pagac and Lieneke (LEE-na-ka) Hafeman. In this chapter, I summarize their comments about nursing education, students, and faculty. Their comments ferried me more deeply into the nursing education undertow and, as a result, additional personal reflections have come to light.

Two reactions surfaced as I first heard Krystle and Lieneke's remarks. First, I sensed their penetrating insight about nursing education, dedication to its importance, and grasp of the challenges for students and faculty. Second, I must admit, I found myself jumping to explain, to excuse, and to defend what we do as teachers and how we do it. As I sat on my hands and bit my tongue, the students' discernment and wisdom about the teaching-learning process astonished me and I became evermore convinced that most other students likely share a similar understanding. I also remembered the countless times in the past when I *did* explain, excuse, and defend with many other students. In those instances, I should have spoken less and listened more.

I interviewed the two students informally with no plan for research rigor. I hope our casual talk can stimulate a well-designed study, spur further discussion, or at least call each of us educators to whittle a deeper perception of all students. I've made every effort to present the students' opinions and experiences thoroughly and accurately. They also reviewed the chapter to help with this effort. Lieneke and Krystle, on behalf of all nurse educators and nursing students everywhere, please accept our gratitude for your generous time, gifted thinking, and gracious courage to teach.

WHO DO THE STUDENTS SAY THAT THEY ARE?

After the three of us warmed up to each other, we began where I thought was a sound place to start: Who are the students? Lieneke and Krystle candidly described themselves and their student nurse colleagues. They playfully shared a few observations and both nodded in agreement with a swaggering smile, "This is just how we are."

As expected, the students immediately identified their stress in learning nursing: "Nursing is always changing, there is a past, present, and a future. . . . There is so much detail . . . and we try to learn it all." They perceived nursing to be different from other disciplines and believed that its overwhelming nature is a key factor in their stress.

The students' description of their stress puzzles me; in fact, student stress has troubled me for a long time. It seems that there is more to the students' stress than the nature of nursing itself. Even though they fervently engage in nursing as a career, why are so many students "so sick of school" by the time they complete their first degree? As educators, are we increasingly more stressed and therefore fueling the students' stress? Why are so few students interested in nursing education? Do they see us and not like what they see? As the nursing body of knowledge grows, do we simply add more facts and multiply the content, continuing to teach exactly as we were taught? Or is there a power factor that shapes our relationships with students in distressing ways or in ways that we may not see or care to admit?

In addition to living the stress of learning nursing, Lieneke and Krystle were quick to point out that nursing students also are unique. Nursing students feel pressured and are "extraordinarily motivated, obsessive-compulsive, anal, worried about doing the best we can, and we question everything." The students admitted that their competition is strong: "We don't lose competitiveness as we move through the program . . . we always care a lot about our grade, even after we are admitted and assured of a spot." They view feedback incredibly seriously and long remember its detail. Being part of a cohort where relationships build over several years, as well as having "a nursing building, classrooms, and labs where we come together," buffers the students' anxiety and builds their resilience.

So, this is who the students say they are. In our interview, we continued with additional basics—fundamental, but equally priceless.

THE NURSE EDUCATOR: WHAT IS MOST IMPORTANT?

I then asked Krystle and Lieneke, "What are the most important things for you about the nursing faculty?" Their opinions poured out quickly and freely, twisting and turning as they reinforced each other. The students knew precisely what mattered to them about the professors: knowing the content, enthusiasm, consistency, organization, and positive regard for students.

Familiarity with the Content

First, the students saw teachers' familiarity with the content as essential. This familiarity enabled faculty to "filter out what's important." When teachers know the content, they can be concise, emphasize key points, and use examples and their own nursing experiences to "help us remember."

I have had many students and alumni retell me semesters or years later the textured details of an experience I shared in class to highlight an idea I was teaching. Needless to say, I have long forgotten the incidents, but the students remember. They recall learning about deontology as an ethical theory linked with the story of my dying hospitalized father asking for tomato juice (which was denied). They also remember learning about nursing interventions at the end of life when I moved the heart rhythm display off the bedside monitor so that a family could stop staring at the screen and redirect their attention to their dying mother lying in her bed.

The students remember my stories. Just as I still remember Miss Mary Lewis, one of my OB instructors when I was a nursing student in the early 1970s. She disclosed her experiences distributing birth control items and information as she clung to the back of a motorcycle driven by one of the local Catholic priests. Of course, this prompted a spirited in- and out-of-class discussion about birth control methods and availability, religious beliefs, and rebellion . . . ah, those were the seventies. Miss Lewis certainly knew the content she was teaching and used her own entertaining experiences to sharply underscore key points, showcase their intricacy, and help us remember.

Krystle and Lieneke have experienced numerous class presentations given by faculty obviously unfamiliar with the content; "those professors basically summarized the textbook, with no other examples. . . . We could have done that without coming to class." When the teachers know the content and help students see the "must know" points, it prevents teachers from "leaving content for us to do on our own outside of class." Both students detested when significant content was not reviewed in class. Other students in the past have told me that when a professor frequently leaves substantial amounts of content for them "to do on our own," the students perceive this as faculty disorganization, content unfamiliarity, or even laziness. "The professors dealt with their own 'not knowing' by just leaving it for us to do—then they themselves don't have to learn it."

For a nurse educator to know the content seems obvious. It's splendid when we teach content that's familiar to us or that we've experienced. But how can we manage when that is not the case—when we're teaching chronic illnesses in children, for instance, and have never practiced a single day in pediatric service?

In my first year as an educator, I was assigned to teach the care of burn patients to senior students in a community college in southern California. I never saw a hospitalized burn patient in my life and only dimly remembered a few foggy shreds from my own nursing education. Although tempting because I had absolutely no specialized details or experiences at my fingertips, I couldn't bear to leave the students learn this content on their own. After my jitters settled, I read voraciously about burn patients, distilled the content common to the majority of readings, and disregarded most of the details.

Using those commonalities, I decided to build on what the students already knew well: normal skin functions (i.e., protective barrier against infection, role in balancing body fluids, temperature control, and presence of sensory receptors). Furthermore, from other diseases the students also knew about infection, fluid and electrolyte balance, and pain management, which were key areas in the care of burn patients. My teaching, then, was not a summary of the two assigned textbook chapters but was organized around (1) how the skin's healthy functions are pathologically changed by the burn and (2) how the medical and nursing care are similar or different from situations the students already learned (e.g., preventing and managing infection, maintaining fluid and electrolyte balance).

Admittedly, we did not review every detail about burn patients (as a nurse educator with significant experience in this area could have done), but the students left the class understanding five or six basic processes that occur in burn patients and how to help manage them. In this way, I was using my expertise as a nurse in medical-surgical and cardiac intensive care to filter out what's important and emphasize major points. Also, we all practiced one aspect of constructivist learning; that is, we practiced learning by building on what we know.

Besides reading widely to prepare for this teaching, I also arranged to spend a day with an expert nurse in a burn unit in a nearby city. With that nurse, I studied patients with different burn classifications, in different stages of recovery, and in various emotional and family response systems. That day I also experienced the "culture" of the burn unit: how nurses collaborate with each other, with physicians, and with families, as well as the sights, sounds, and smells of the unit itself. As expected, I had a filled notebook by the end of the day and continued to journal as I sifted through my thoughts and feelings. In that first-time teaching about burn patients, I wove in much of this shadowing experience and discovered how my shadowing brightened and lifted the content, the students, and myself. As I was teaching the burn content, I also sensed the confidence and skill of that expert nurse in the classroom with me.

Since that first year of teaching, I have shadowed numerous other nurses, such as a home healthcare nurse working with homebound indigent clients and an IV team nurse working extensively with central intravenous lines, to gain familiarity with specific content. All of these times were invaluable because I had the luxury of just watching, listening, and asking questions. I had no responsibility for clinical students accompanying me or accountability to provide patient care. I find that my shadowing experiences are more robust if I read substantially in preparation—they are my essential professional development, my scholarship of discovery.

If I may digress here, I'd like to slip in just a word about networking. A ho-hum, overused term perhaps, but I have learned the immeasurable worth of deliberately establishing and graciously maintaining connections with a wide array of individuals in the healthcare system. As precious as any professional journal, textbook, or Web site, my off-campus colleagues continually serve as e-mail and telephone resources, arrange "shadowings" for me and dozens of interested students, and provide me with consultant and advisory opportunities. Those colleagues have warmly opened their doors and offered the skill of their staff to help us learn. In return, I've presented staff development sessions, shared firsthand information about our nursing education programs, and served as an occasional coach or mentor (this service is one of my most relished teaching rewards).

I cannot overemphasize the value of this networking. Actually, the network itself has been one of my own mentors. In the literature, *mentor* refers to an individual person, but in my case this network, this group of colleagues in the practice setting, has been my mentor. I encourage new faculty to begin these relationships immediately and intentionally—face to face, in writing, through participation in professional organizations, at the kids' soccer games, and in all other ways possible. Connections may begin with a nursing director on a hospital unit, an earlier acquaintance who is now a staff nurse in an area

steady expectations: for example, format for writing the literature review in their paper, use of first or third person, and type and minimum number of references. Vague faculty responses to the students' questions about assignment details, such as "just write a scholarly paper" or "make sure it's written at a college level," aggravate the students. The students admitted that sometimes "we just throw our hands up in despair . . . not really caring what happens . . . it can become a 'we' versus 'they' situation." This definitely sounds out of rhythm.

I often hear annoyed faculty "diss-ing" students for asking these detail questions about the assignment: "Can't they figure it out? They should be using the APA manual. They're so worried about the little things." Yet these "little things" become "bigger things" as points are deducted on the paper grade, which, not surprisingly, further escalates the students' irritation.

These uncertainties and unanswered questions about a course assignment hinder the students. Early in my teaching career I also believed that students could figure it out. They should be individual and unique in their writing and I didn't want to impose any rules. The details didn't really matter to me (but I realized that they did matter when I was grading the papers).

Delineating the major paper format items (those that are important to me) in the course syllabus or in written assignment guidelines saves time and worry. I simply list them in bullet fashion (in writing so that they can serve as an ongoing reference). For example: (1) approximate length of paper 6–8 pages, (2) needs intro, body, and conclusion, (3) must have a thesis or purpose statement, (4) first or third person is acceptable, (5) level I headings are essential, and the like. Until the students are clear about these details, their frustrations spiral up and prevent critical engagement with the intended content. I also outline in writing and discuss in class how their papers need to be individualized and unique (e.g., showing how to build on another general education [GE] class, link with their family, or compare to a recent movie they've seen). That is, the paper uniqueness is not in the general format but in the substantive developed content.

Consistency also refers to a longer term relationship with one faculty in the course. In the program, there are numerous team-taught courses with five to seven teachers in one course, perhaps each teaching a week or two of classes in the semester. Krystle and Lieneke unmistakably described their wish for a smaller number of faculty so that consistency was stronger.

Last, consistency is important from a classroom teaching perspective. The students insisted that when they're familiar with a certain teacher, they can listen more closely, take notes easily, and connect with more of the details. "I'm not spending so much time and energy figuring out where the teacher is going . . . going fast in class is okay, because it's the same pattern . . . when I know what to expect, I learn more, I'm less worried." Several approaches help students know what to expect, such as (1) listing major points for the class time on the blackboard, on the first PowerPoint slide, or under the document camera, (2) using a written class handout that outlines the presentation, and (3) occasional pauses in class (or between class meetings) identifying "where we've been and where we need to go." In my early years as a teacher, I felt this type of listing or outline or review was excessive, even pointless. I just assumed the students knew where things were going; after all, I was crystal clear in my own lecture notes and in my own thoughts. Since then, however, I've learned that any lucidity I can provide for the students functions as signpost, as framework, as the string holding the beads together.

Students also crave consistency as they prepare for exams: "With fewer teachers, I know how to study for the exams; I could almost predict what's going to be on the test, even guessing some of the wording in the test questions."

Now I'm beginning to understand what it means to "get a rhythm with a teacher." It seems to be all the things we do with students that enhance clarity and predictability, providing a focus and details as they are needed—yet not strangling any of our energy and liveliness.

Organization surfaced as a fourth crucial element of being a nurse educator: organized syllabus at the start of the semester, with major units, readings, due dates, and out-of-class activities clearly presented. When these main course components continuously change or trickle in, week in and week out over the semester, the students waste time and energy sorting out the bedlam. Conversely, when faculty are organized in the course, Lieneke unflinchingly related: "We can feel their relaxation . . . and we can relax ourselves . . . and when we're relaxed, we can learn more." However, organization was also treasured as a balance with spontaneity. Krystle recalled a history class where there was less structure, more story- and experience telling, and a more relaxed atmosphere; yet, "we learned tons about the history content." This could "probably work in nursing," she solemnly submitted.

I staggered and stumbled, reeling in my own thoughts. This could "probably work in nursing"? Why *doesn't* this happen in nursing? Why *aren't* we paying attention to the students' relaxation and their worry? Why *aren't* we drawing on our experiences to help students learn and remember? The students bravely tell us, and we know when someone worries less and relaxes more, learning escalates.

Relationships with Students

Lieneke and Krystle stood firm on the final point: How faculty view students is a key element of being a nurse educator. Without any doubts, they pinpointed several examples they found indispensable. Being respected as a student and treated as an adult are paramount. In their respect, the faculty "give us options for an assignment . . . they really want us to succeed and will work with us so we don't fail . . . we can talk with most any professor." Notably, one of the students felt more respected in some of her nonnursing classes.

The students further described faculty approachability and accessibility. First, the hallway vibe is significant. "It's easy to tell if the faculty vibe is 'I don't want to be bothered.' But if the vibe is positive and friendly in the hallway, five weeks later when I need help, that is the professor I will approach." Second, the students treasure office presence. "The professors are physically in their office which is often more helpful than a quick response on e-mail . . . e-mail is great, but sometimes I really need to sit and talk."

For me, maintaining office presence has been a challenging dilemma. Without a doubt, there is the faculty continuum from "never there" to "almost always there." Although I've been criticized for "pampering or spoiling the students" by being too available, I remain steadfast in my belief in the worth of office presence.

I try to be in my office more often than not, especially around class times. I feel the merit in those thousands of times when students hesitate in the doorway and then ask courteously, "Do you have just a minute?" or "This will only take a couple minutes." And in those precious minutes, which usually become a half hour or even an hour, the teaching and learning premiums happen. The students and I answer questions, reframe problems, review tests, explore futures, generate ideas, share stories, and make referrals. In those office minutes, students are upheld, kinship is shaped, rhythm is practiced, and I am continually inspired—in a way that rarely happens in the classroom.

Students frequently stop by my office when they are somewhere in the mid-stages of writing a paper. With helter-skelter pages, arrows circling about their paragraphs, and a plea in their eyes, the need seems urgent because I suspect the student will be spending the next 4 to 5 hours working on the paper. I can quickly review a thesis statement, check headings and sections of the paper for organization and content development, examine quality of references, verify an intro, body, and conclusion, and highlight any other needed format changes.

In this could-you-just-look-at-my-paper office stop, students typically need the most help with the content that is not a summary of the literature, such as the connection with a specific GE class they've taken or link with a client population. Going beyond summarizing the literature seems most challenging for students and often turns out to be more superficial and vague. Posing specific questions about GE interest areas and suggesting ideas for the student to consider is often all that is needed. For example, "You told me you've been learning about foot binding in 19th-century China in your Asian History class. What connection can you describe between this practice and the clients you are working with at the Refuge House for battered women?"

I would much rather help students develop ideas further and polish in draft form than mark all of this on the final paper. For me, face-to-face communication at the "office stop" during the paper-writing process is more efficient and helpful than electronic communication. In this office-stop dialogue, the student and I respond to each other immediately and I can clarify, illustrate with more examples, notice nonverbals, and simply show how. Naturally, I provide all the positive feedback that is possible, such as affirming the topic choice and the thorough development of a key point. As a result of this early review, the paper is stronger, there has been an opportunity to revise, the students feel more encouraged, and my time is more effectively used.

At other times, a student may stop by for more than one reason. I remember when Dahlia came to my office to review the items she missed on a recent test. I was a little perplexed because she scored well. My antenna went up, and fortunately, I put my next meeting on the back burner even though I knew it was convening in about 3 minutes. Something just didn't seem right. We finished the test review, but the conversation hung in midair.

Prompted slightly, Dahlia painfully described her life as a first-generation college student (although she did not call it that). She perceived herself to be living two lives. The first was a stimulating, thrilling life on campus where she successfully achieved her academic goals and met interesting and different people. The second was a "dragged down" life at home where her parents and siblings ridiculed her for not staying home and "getting a real job where she could make money rather than spend it." Dahlia shyly admitted, "They have no idea what my life is like . . . they don't really know me . . . we don't even speak the same way anymore."

Dahlia's story is analogous to many other first-generation college students' experiences. In *Lipstick Jihad*, Azadeh Moaveni (2005) describes her own Iranian-American young life in northern California, which she calls a "hyphenated life"—another example of trying to navigate two worlds. "There was Azadeh at school, who managed to look and sound like the other kids, barring the occasional lunchbox oddity; and there was Azadeh at home, who lived in a separate world, with its own special language and rituals . . . living between two cultures just made me long for refuge in one" (p. 19).

As Dahlia and I discussed at length the first-generation experience, I hoped to normalize what she was feeling. I wrote down the name and phone number of one of the university counselors who worked extensively with first-generation students and gave it to her. I've learned that names and contact information given to the student in writing sends a more serious message and has longer staying power than verbal information. Later in the course, Dahlia analyzed the first-generation experience, relating her own life, the counselor's discussion, and a wide body of literature in a brilliant paper.

Looking back, I'm relieved I did not rush away to my other meeting that day when Dahlia stopped by for a minute to look at her test. I know there were many times with many students that I did dash off, but I hope those times resulted in few serious consequences and I offer my deepest apologies for the times I should have stayed.

In order to help keep myself as fully available as possible when I am in my office, I also try to schedule chunks of time away from my office to work on other scholarship activities. Most semesters I'm able to accomplish that and I've learned that writing this in my calendar helps me stay with the plan. For example, when I write "library" or "research" every Wednesday from 12–5 p.m. I'm more likely to adhere to the plan. This approach helps me move my schol-arship forward and also be less dependent on my office presence time for these responsibilities. Of course, there have been times that I've needed to postpone meeting with a student because of another commitment I could not rearrange. And if truth be told, I've never been able to adhere to rigorously scheduled office hours—I seem to get distracted or involved in the day's work and the office hour structure burdens me. When all is said and done, perhaps each instructor needs to design a workable, accessible, and significant way to be present with students outside of the classroom, for it is that presence that is one of the teaching ultimates.

For Krystle and Lieneke, then, and probably for the majority of other stu-dents, fine nursing education calls for a teacher who knows the content, knows how to teach it with energy and commitment to the students' learning, and can blend organization with spontaneity. This teacher is summoned to be authen-tically student-centered and recognize that teaching and learning and kinship happen in all different ways and in diverse places. Finally, consistency among faculty within a course and maximum clarity about faculty expectations sustain an effective educational experience. When all these dimensions come together, learning skyrockets and students are challenged and liberated when they relax more, worry less, and "get a rhythm with the teacher."

ABOUT BEING A *NEW* NURSE EDUCATOR

"And now, what about being a new faculty? What advice do you have for new teachers?" Lieneke and Krystle looked at each other, with sparkle and warm smiles: "Just tell new teachers that experience will help, . . . and tell them also that they won't be able to reach all of the students all of the time." I sensed the students' gentleness and encouragement and also suspect that they intimately related to being novices themselves, as they too slid and slipped into a new nursing role.

To start, these two students emphatically counseled new faculty to know themselves, recognizing that everyone's personality is different. Knowing themselves, they said about new faculty, results in their ability to honestly and fully say, "This is how I am."

With no intent to offend, Lieneke and Krystle gracefully described the emotions they observed in new faculty. They identified new teachers' anxiety and unease, depicted their affect as sometimes flat in the classroom, and often discerned little excitement in the new faculty about the content they are teaching. New teachers' discomfort unmistakably affects the students: "We know they're nervous, but it makes us frustrated if they don't know where they're going in the content. Sometimes they go too fast in class because they're so nervous." They also saw new faculty as either over- or underconfident: "They expect us to be experts and they don't realize how much work they're expecting . . . or sometimes they think we don't know anything."

By and large, students forgive, support, and are patient with new faculty, although on occasion this is not the case. A disconnect, an out-of-rhythm relationship, or even hostility between the students and the new teacher can shackle learning, disgrace the students, and crush the faculty. In view of that possibility, what can new teachers do so that students will work with them rather than against them?

First, honesty balanced with confidence supports a buoyant learning environment. Acknowledging one's newness (which the students will know on day 1) and then moving on seems most useful. I've heard new faculty continually remind students that "I'm new at this," or "I've never done this content before," or "You're my guinea pigs," or "Now that I've bored you to death," or even "Don't pay much attention to what I'm saying." (Incidentally, we would never say this as a novice nurse working with clients, so why do we keep repeating this with students?) This continual or even infrequent reminder only weakens the new teacher's skill, damages the students' perception of the new faculty, and erodes trust. After all, if the teacher doesn't believe in herself or himself, why should the students? And students tire of hearing the "I'm new" mantra because their emphasis is on learning the course content and linking it with their professional and personal lives.

Second, new faculty must admit mistakes (but not dwell on them) and be flexible. In my early years of teaching, I rarely changed a due date for a course assignment, altered a grade, or dropped a test item because the students were confused or thought it unfair or that I had written it poorly. At that time, I didn't want to be perceived as "waffly" or uncertain. I've now learned that accommodating student requests based on their solid, documented, and convincing rationale is much healthier. In this way, the students practice negotiating and using their voice, which is an essential skill as a nurse and a citizen, and they are also more respectful and understanding when their requests are denied. For me, this approach creates a more collaborative culture and I feel more liberated in the educator role; that is, the students are invited to make requests of me and I also am free to make requests of them.

I've also discovered, although this took me several years, that I almost always wait a day or two before making a decision about a student's major request. I try to minimize the "we/they" attitude by saying, "Thank you, I really appreciate you asking, your request is significant, and I need to take a day to think about it. I will consider it very seriously and get back to you at our next class." Buying time gives me an opportunity to read the students' rationale and think more carefully and thoroughly rather than deciding on the spot in front of 50 or 100 eager and watchful pairs of eyes.

Krystle and Lieneke also suggested specific "do's and don'ts" for both new and experienced educators. Their comments centered on use of PowerPoint, as well as course assignments and the feedback they received.

PowerPoint is most effective when key words or phrases are presented on the slides, not "single random words which are too vague." They cautioned that teachers must then expand those key points with discussion, experiences, and meaningful details. Again, the students adamantly endorsed their need to learn "between the lines"—the stories and additions to help them understand and remember. Using an accompanying paper handout of the PowerPoint is beneficial "if the print is large enough with adequate space for my notes." PowerPoint is least effective when the faculty merely read the words on the slide and "this goes on slide after slide."

Course assignments invited a lively interchange in our interview. The students loathe course activities that are "busy work . . . it's just so tedious and boring." They also abhor "tons of reading. If there is too much, we just don't do any of it. Smaller, designated page numbers are more manageable." Students appreciate when faculty identify important readings: "Most of the time we can't tell what's important and what is merely 'nice to know.'" Of course, teachers must be familiar with the content to prioritize readings, differentiating between required and recommended.

The students also noted the extensive amounts of writing in their nursing classes: "These huge scholarly papers seem to be overkill, especially if we have several in each of our nursing classes during the same semester." Thinking more is better, educators often loosely assign one giant scholarly paper on the heels of another; maybe we need to reshape writing assignments to achieve specific writing outcomes. Additionally, journaling generated mixed student responses. Although journaling "helps us understand our patients," often journals are "basically busywork." Finally, the students valued preparing a self-evaluation as part of a course assignment because it enhanced their learning and prepared them for professional practice. "We know there will always be a next time and nurses self-evaluate all the time."

Interestingly, Lieneke and Krystle also preferred classroom meetings rather than Web-based teaching. In addition, they appreciated when faculty used only one communication approach. Some professors use multiple communication channels, such as Web-based instruction, e-mail, and verbal or written communication. In these situations, the students found themselves inefficiently checking multiple places so that they wouldn't miss anything; sometimes the messages in each were slightly different, which multiplied the confusion.

Finally, feedback was enormously important to the students. Receiving a grade only or a cursory comment was not helpful. Lieneke noted emphatically, "I must know, does the teacher understand the idea that I'm writing?" Krystle concurred, "I need to learn what I can do differently . . . and how to do that."

Over the years, students have often discussed the benefit of feedback. One student reported that "Great Paper-A" was all a professor wrote on the last page of her 40-page paper. She regretted the absence of feedback: "How was I to know what was strong about the paper and what I could change? I spent days writing the paper and it seemed like it was nearly a waste of my time." Do we forget that providing feedback is teaching and that it fosters learning?

Almost unbelievably, I had another student tell me that she somehow fixed the pages on her paper so that she could determine whether the pages had been opened and turned. She suspected the teacher was not reading the students' papers but only writing a grade on the last page. Using this tactic (I did not ask for any details), the student was nearly positive her paper had not been read and yet she received an A written on the very last page. You can imagine how this discovery shocked the student (and how the grapevine shrieked with this finding).

For new faculty, then, what is the take-home message from Krystle and Lieneke's remarks? Three principal suggestions emerged: (1) teaching requires practice, (2) self-reflection is essential, and (3) specific strategies, such as course assignments and providing feedback, demand careful and methodical scrutiny because they propel students' energy and learning.

BEYOND BALANCE

I'd like to return to this chapter's first paragraph where I proposed a balance between the faculty perspective and the student perspective. I'm changing my mind. As I listened to Krystle and Lieneke's comments, wrote this chapter, and deliberated the balance idea more intensely—I now would like to offer a slightly different angle.

A balance between the faculty and student perspective, as I first suggested, tautly outlines a polarity, a rival divergence, voices in opposite corners of the classroom. Where the faculty lounge in one end of the building and the students congregate down another hallway (and rarely the two shall meet), it is nearly impossible to deny the polarity, the isolation. There is no wonder that many of these same students continue as alumni to huddle in their breakrooms and cafeteria corners of the healthcare system, unable to come to the collaboration and problem-solving tables in their practice settings. And it is no wonder that they often are incapable of inspiring or affecting decisions that matter. Might it be that we've become too comfortable, too consensual in this segregation—in this "balance"? The students have learned their lesson well, although I mourn the result.

Instead, I suggest that students and faculty are related, and they are parts of a single whole. They are inseparable, reciprocal. As Rico (2000) submits, "In order to know one, you must know the other . . . one side only exists in relationship to the other" (p. 193). It is not either/or but *both* students *and* faculty. We must design ways to live, to learn, and to teach that are complementary. We must bring faculty and students out of their respective lounges, physically and metaphorically, to circle a more shared table.

REFERENCES

Beck, M. N. (1999). *Expecting Adam: A story of birth, rebirth, and everyday magic.* New York: Times Books.

Coetzee, J. M. (2005). *Slow man.* New York: Viking Penguin.

Moaveni, A. (2005). *Lipstick jihad: A memoir of growing up Iranian in America and American in Iran.* New York: Perseus Books Group.

Rico, G. (2000). *Writing the natural way: Using right-brain techniques to release your expressive powers.* New York: Penguin Putnam.

CHAPTER 7

Presence with Students: Posing Interest, Not Merely Paying Attention

I Taught Them All

I have taught high school for 10 years. During that time, I have given assignments, among others, to a murderer, an evangelist, a pugilist, a thief, and an imbecile.

The murderer was a quiet little boy who sat on the front seat and regarded me with pale blue eyes; the evangelist, easily the most popular boy in school, had the lead in the junior play; the pugilist lounged by the window and let loose at intervals a raucous laugh that startled even the geraniums; the thief was a gay-hearted Lothario with a song on his lips; and the imbecile, a soft-eyed little animal seeking the shadows.

The murderer awaits death in the state penitentiary; the evangelist has lain a year now in the village churchyard; the pugilist lost an eye in a brawl in Hong Kong; the thief, by standing on tiptoe, can see the windows of my room from the county jail; and the once gentle-eyed little moron beats his head against a padded wall in the state asylum.

All of these pupils once sat in my room, sat and looked at me gravely across worn brown desks. I must have been a great help to those pupils— I taught them the rhyming scheme of the Elizabethan sonnet and how to diagram a complex sentence.

—Naomi White

Alice's family heaped piles of *attention* on her, yet she was the heir of no one's *interest*.

Joyce Carol Oates (2003) describes Alice James living in a time when "girls seem scarcely to have had a chance" (p. 65). Alice was the younger sister of William and Henry, sons of a wealthy intellectual family; one was an internationally renowned psychologist–philosopher and the other an author. Diagnosed with breast cancer at age 43, Alice "lies on her couch forever," a "victim of fainting spells, convulsions, fits of hysteria, mysterious paralyzing pains, and such nineteenth-century female maladies as nervous hyperesthesia, spinal neurosis, cardiac complication, and rheumatic gout . . . she does not matter in the public world, in the world of men, of history. She does not count; she *is* nothing" (p. 66).

In her career-invalidism, Alice's family admittedly paid considerable *attention* to her, but no one posed any *interest*. That is, her health problems received attention. Although this attending likely was mechanical, even aloof, family members did look after her daily faints, minister to her paralyzing pains, and wait on her "forever couch."

Despite the automated attention she received, Alice did not count and she did not matter. If someone had posed interest in her, it would have gone beyond her tribulations and miseries and made Alice count. By posing interest, her psychologist brother William would have viewed her as a human being rather than studying her as a "collection of symptoms." Posing interest does not merely attend to her predicament—posing interest unites with Alice and who she is.

In a comparable way, posing *interest* with students is vastly different from paying *attention*. How we establish presence is a critical part of teaching, and yet we frequently overlook it.

Perhaps we assume that simply bringing students and faculty together in higher education instinctively creates a meaningful presence with students. Might it be that we pay attention to student-centeredness in education, but we pose little interest in students? Might it be that we view students, but we don't encounter them, we don't unite with them? In this chapter, I invite you to contemplate posing interest in students in both clinical and classroom teaching by showing up, circulating, and getting inside the students' heads.

Naomi White taught sentence diagramming and the rhyming schemes of Elizabethan sonnets to the murderer, evangelist, pugilist, thief, and imbecile. In her remembering, she begs us to ponder the paying attention or posing interest question. Of course, it is preposterous to assume that one or the other was or was not occurring in her teaching.

Unmistakably, however, White directs us to pose interest in the nursing students sitting in our classrooms. In addition to dutifully listing the sonnets and sentences in our syllabus, we must hear White's wise and far-sighted mandate to pose interest in the nursing students who look at us "gravely across worn brown desks," search for us earnestly across online courses, and hunt for us desperately in the mess and madness of our healthcare system. For one day we too will be summoned to admit that we have "taught them all."

POSING INTEREST AS A CLINICAL TEACHER: AN EARLY LESSON

As educators, we must amplify the specific needs of individual students and not solely extrapolate from educational theories—we must pose interest, not merely pay attention. To pose interest is to affirm, encourage, acknowledge, sustain, support, and encounter.

An experience I had as a novice clinical instructor shattered my complacency around attention versus interest. As obvious as this seems, it was a difficult lesson for me and took several years to learn. In fact, a couple of clinical students who tweaked up their fortitude during a postclinical conference were my early teachers. At that time, I did not recognize students' need for and response to affirmation, to the teacher posing interest.

I demanded high clinical performance from the first day the students tensely stepped off the elevator and onto the clinical unit. This was a time when I wrongly expected excellence immediately, not realizing, of course, that clinical experiences are a time for learning and not only a time for evaluation. At the end of a postclinical conference, well into the 8-week hospital rotation, one valiant voice asked me, "Why don't you ever tell us when we do well?" She formed each word reluctantly and framed each syllable in an "I'm a courteous Midwesterner" accent.

I wanted to die. I could not have felt more crushed, more deflated. I was certain that I would be the perfect teacher. Up to that time, I had not heard anything like this directly from students, or from anyone else, for that matter. That day, however, I heard the student's question shrieking that I was light-years away from perfect. My ego's strewn splinters covered the floor while the students' downward gazes deadened the silence. As my face beefed crimson, I tried to recover and stumbled out something coldly academic like "you need to know that you are doing well, unless I call your attention to something specific." Another bold student gingerly piped up, "But we need to *hear* from you that *we are doing okay.*" Oh, let the plucky students come!

From that day forward, I deliberated about posing interest, not merely paying attention. For me, to authentically affirm, acknowledge, encourage, support, and sustain, I had to learn more deeply about the students.

As I said, authentic affirmation did not come easily. Although I was affirmed by many of my own teachers, positive comments were in short supply in my family home. Except for my father's frequent dignified encouragement, I rarely remember hearing anyone in my home tell me that I was doing well, or what I could do differently to do well.

In learning about authentic affirmation in clinical teaching, it may have helped me to also delve into the characters of Jane Austen's *Pride and Prejudice.* Since that novice teaching experience, I've learned about the role of voice and dialogue in the novel: the wide variety of verbal and written discourse within and between people. It is as if the dialogue creates and settles all the strains. Further, I've come to appreciate that the most heartless characters in many of Austen's novels are those who are incapable of an authentic, two-way discourse—those characters only lecture, fume, and seethe.

Studying Austen's work, and other novelists, I'm sure, would have helped me pause and self-reflect on my own interaction style. Using another medium in this way to look inside is what Palmer (2004) calls studying one's self "on the slant . . . giving my shy soul the protective cover it needs" (pp. 92–93). He maintains that sometimes looking directly at the self is too sharp, maybe too fierce. Similar to some of Austen's characters, perhaps I too needed to move beyond one-way talk and closer to two-way dialogue.

Making heartening comments to students about their capable performance initially felt twisted, unnatural, and unnecessary. But gradually, as the result of a beginning two-way dialogue, I was able to say: (1) "Jill, the discharge teaching you did with that patient was very good—you repeated major points, included his wife in your discussion, verified that he understood, and incorporated health literacy guidelines," (2) "You did a great job with your change-of-shift report, Michael—you highlighted significant events from last night, organized your information logically, included key physical and psychosocial items, summarized new medical orders, and did not repeat unnecessary data," and (3) "Shannon, you have a great understanding of how the electrolyte levels and medications are linked together in your patient with congestive heart failure."

Providing sustaining and specific comments slowly crept inside me, as the paint becomes part of the painter's hand. Continuing to hear the value this has for students, I am affirmed in turn and realize that I too need to hear from students that I am doing okay. I also need others to pose interest in me.

POSING INTEREST AS A CLASSROOM TEACHER

Just as it is in clinical teaching, posing interest is also a vital part of classroom teaching. Moreover, posing interest with a *group* of students is just as decisive as posing interest with an *individual*. I had a recent experience that illuminated the essence of posing interest with an entire class.

A seasoned faculty colleague who has been working diligently on her teaching skills asked me to visit one of her class lectures to provide feedback on her teaching. Celeste (not her real name) and I have been friends for many years, so I welcomed this comfortable invitation. Four weeks into the semester, I attended Celeste's 2-hour class about the endocrine system with 40 first-semester juniors. Because this was a team-taught course, this was the first time that semester when Celeste was actually in front of the students teaching the class.

Celeste and I were able to follow up my visit to her class with an open and honest dialogue. As is often true in those kinds of conversations, we both uncovered more deeply how we teach and what we learn.

I did what I could to help Celeste appreciate the fact that recognizing the level of most of the students' knowledge—seeing the overall class perception—is an essential component of posing interest. In her class, the students' understanding of the endocrine system demonstrated several characteristics where the concept of a "nudge," as proposed by Thaler and Sunstein (2008), may be helpful. With backgrounds in economics, behavioral science, and jurisprudence, Thaler and Sunstein describe nudging as designing or organizing the context in which people make decisions, especially in complex situations and situations that occur infrequently, where mistakes are likely. Although their focus is on decisions related to health, wealth, and happiness, applying the nudge notion to education might open up several possibilities to help us pose interest. Celeste's lesson on the endocrine system was a perfect opportunity to provide students a nudge because the endocrine system is *complex*, detailed encounters with it may be *infrequent* for some students, and there tends to be a higher rate of *error* in comprehending it.

First, I suggested that the context could be designed so that there would be less teacher talking about endocrine minutiae and more student talking about major ideas linked to actual patient situations. Nudging students to understand the endocrine system by emphasizing main points and fundamental ideas, and then helping students learn to apply them is another dimension of posing interest.

For example, rather than lecturing about every single action of all the glands and hormones in the endocrine system, it may be more meaningful to analyze a case study. For example, a 12-year-old boy with type 1 diabetes who develops a wound infection and acute renal disease after a car accident. Consistent with Thaler and Sunstein's (2008) nudging in a wide array of life situations, nudging in this way can make the information more comprehensible, transform key points into actual use, and provide immediate feedback.

Recall my unrealistic expectations for expertise and perfection the moment students begin their clinical experience. In the same way, I have found that classroom educators fresh from a veteran staff nurse or nurse practitioner role frequently teach and expect the same sophisticated level of understanding, application, and detail from beginning students. These unexamined assumptions about students' knowledge and skill may prevent us from truly seeing the overall class awareness level and, therefore, prevent us from posing interest.

Second, noticing Celeste's students' confusion around the class handout, I suggested a simpler version. Again, simplifying the handout would nudge students to understand major ideas related to the endocrine system. Much too much content was crammed vertically and horizontally onto about three pages, with small print and detailed, slightly fuzzy drawings of feedback loops with arrows. This handout needed to be downsized by (1) selecting essential key points, (2) opening up some white space, (3) enlarging the drawings and the font size, and (4) paraphrasing rather than cut and pasting the textbook details.

As always, I was edified by Celeste's dedication to classroom teaching and the students' commitment to learn the course content. They knew it was critical to their own nursing practice, and of course they knew it would be on the test. As the class period unfolded, however, students' anxiety bubbled up with growing panicky whispering and handout highlighting.

Reflecting back, I realize I probably wasn't very helpful to Celeste. I assume that she made some of the changes I suggested, or perhaps she didn't. I also expect that the following semester around week 4, when the endocrine content came up again, the same anxiety bubbled and the same panic whispered.

My "ah-ha" of this experience is that Celeste's connection with students happened a long time before she taught her class on the endocrine system in week 4 of the semester. Degrees of posing interest and paying attention had been etched in how the relationship was crafted. As Jane Austen's characters teach us, we need to consider to what extent an authentic, two-way dialogue was generated.

Celeste's relationship with the students had already long been established before week 4. Perhaps the relationship began with the tone of the syllabus, that is, how the rules were presented, Celeste's approach to test make-ups, attendance, paper rewrites, and due dates. More basically, how organized and user-friendly was the syllabus? If the students are frustrated as they try to decipher the syllabus to fill their own planners with the semester's work, the student–teacher relationship is already fraught with reservation, perhaps distrust. Further, what choices do the students have about written assignments, readings, textbooks, topics for papers, and small group organizations?

In these first encounters with the teacher, the students cleverly distinguish the attention they've been paid from the interest that has been posed. If the focus is school—*attention* to rules, regulations, procedures, and so forth— rather than education—*interest* in learning—it is likely that students will feel more constricted in asking questions, admitting confusion, or requesting different teaching methods. My experience has been that occasionally the focus on *attention* actually promotes students' irritation and aggravation.

As I look back on my experience with Celeste, I can see that variations of paying attention and posing interest were already established before the fourth week of the semester. I was undoubtedly "late to class."

SHOWING UP AND CIRCULATING

Whether in clinical or classroom teaching, presence is determined by affirming communication with students, by being with them, learning who they

are. Our teaching cannot be ruled only by formal theory, recipes, and techniques. Our teaching cannot be dictated by centralized, unyielding policies.
Revealing the merit of presence, Dr. Marjorie Bottoms, one of my faculty
mentor-friends, insisted in her endearing, gallant way that a substantial part of
our responsibility in education as faculty and as students is "just showing up."
But it is the *way* we show up that edges us closer either to posing interest or
just paying attention.

Abraham Lincoln championed showing up throughout his law practice and
presidency (Phillips, 1992). During the Civil War, he spent most of his time
away from 1600 Pennsylvania Avenue as he circulated among the troops. In
contemporary language, this is labeled "roving leadership," being in touch,
managing by wandering around, maybe even working the room.

However we label this circulating, there are many benefits. In Lincoln's
situation, he was able to obtain firsthand knowledge to make crucial decisions
without needing to rely solely on others; interact in a relaxed, less pressured
environment; gather public opinion (Lincoln called these "public opinion
baths"); let others know that he could come among them without fear; and
demonstrate his amiability and commitment, as well as his compassion and
sympathy during hospital visits and at funerals. As he showed up and circulated among the troops, Lincoln was posing interest rather than merely paying
attention.

As educators, how do we "circulate among the troops"? Circulating
resourcefully among students mandates that we imagine. Maxine Greene (1995)
compellingly links imagination with empathy, proclaiming that "imagination is
what, above all, makes empathy possible" (p. 3). She believes that it is imagination that helps one feel into the life of another and that "imagination is as
important in the lives of teachers as it is in the lives of their students" (p. 36).
Without imagination, then, there can be little empathy and the circulating is
hollow, empty—without imagination, we end up merely paying attention.

Posing interest insists that we imagine how students are allowed or admitted onto *our* campuses and into *our* classrooms. Metaphorically speaking, is
there an unlocked front gate, a main door with flags flying and emblems posted
that is generously open to all? Or, in addition to the warmly receptive front gate,
is there also a small curtained gap in the wall through which students must
crouch and hesitantly creep with their heads lowered? Is there a restricted
fissure through which students are admitted only after they have been dis-
sected, pored over, and deemed appropriate by the scrutinizing search?

Assuming academic requirements have been met, at the curtained gap
students still might face the more overt constraints, such as gender, race, and
sexual orientation. And as we imagine more intensely, we unlock the more
covert restrictions with which students tentatively tiptoe into our classrooms:
obesity, military affiliation, atheism, tattoos and body piercing, particular

dialects, hairstyle, dress, or nurse anesthetist as a career goal (which may be sneered at as "not really nursing"). We must admit that we have our own preferences, our own notions of how students should be.

As a result, then, some students may be marginalized and have to work hard to receive our interest. Imagining our own biases and preconceptions—the constraints or restrictions that we present—may be awkward and embarrassing and yet is a key part of posing interest.

There also may be a spectrum in the way we circulate, the way we pose interest or pay attention; that is, it may not be one or the other but a blending of both. Paying attention may be seeing things from afar, through the lens of systems, policy, and success or demographic percentages. For example, we may focus on the retention of first-generation college students or students with excessive numbers of credits at graduation. From this keyhole at a distance, the faces and lives of the students may be veiled. In contrast, posing interest sees things large and up close, such as the details of how students understand, what questions they ask, what silences them, and why they leave. All things considered, in this spectrum we are called to live in both worlds—to live the hyphen between paying attention and posing interest.

As we further examine the concept of circulate, probably most of us declare an open-door policy to help us pose interest. In reality, this policy is far afield from our actual office doors but lives in our e-mail communication, course syllabi, hallway connections with students, walking through learning resource or skills laboratory areas, and written feedback on assignments. One way that I've learned to open the door—to imagine—is to spend more time in the back of the classroom and to sit with students at a study table in the learning resource center. There I learn more about the students, not only seeing what makes them fidget or dull but also what thrills and excites them.

When I circulate I learn that nursing stirs students. Posing interest also means demystifying nursing, helping students learn about nursing on their own so that they can approach the discipline from any slant they choose.

That slant may be a personal experience with cancer, or a sister going public with her homosexuality, or an ambition to link nursing with music. Recently, in an advising meeting in my office, a nursing student who also was a member of the university hockey team and worked as a CNA in a nursing home, shuffled and blushed with embarrassment as she described her interest in gerontology. I'm not sure why I still feel ashamed for her embarrassment. Is it society's ageism that dampened this student's slant? Or was she anticipating a denigrating response from me because of messages I had already sent? Sometimes I also find myself silently chastising a beginning student for choosing nursing as a career because the student simply "wants to help others," as if helping others somehow isn't enough.

Posing interest is helping students find and honor their own slant. But first, of course, we need to inspect our own values, our own rigid reins that we may hold harshly. Nursing cannot be an emotional space or an array of fences and gates that we control to open or close students' learning, their enthusiasm, their personal slant. Students' loyalty to the profession does not exist through us as educators; that is, we cannot hold anything exclusively in our hands as if we are the sanctioned gatekeepers. If we do, we are only paying attention and not posing interest.

I often overhear students' hallway conversations about faculty. I'm always nudged by students' observations and how different those observations are from my own relationship with those very same faculty members. Can those same individuals be so different in our committee meetings or in our course discussions? How is it that these faculty profess to be there for the students and give lip service to being student-centered, when the students' observations are exactly the opposite? Do the students see and hear what I'm not seeing? Am I blind to my colleagues' deeper values and behavior because they are my colleagues, my research partners, my friends? Or is it that the students are astutely discriminating between paying attention and posing interest?

GETTING INSIDE THE STUDENTS' HEADS

Posing interest is getting inside the students' heads. In a keynote address presented in the late 1980s to an organization committed to improving teacher preparation, Dr. Lee Shulman (2004) related what several mathematics educators have repeatedly told their teaching students: "When a child makes a mistake, don't ask 'Why did he do something so stupid?' Get inside that student's head and ask, 'What would make that a *reasonable* thing for him and her to say?'" (p. 413).

Posing interest helps us respond to students' understandings and stumbles. For example, a student may be convinced that the U.S. healthcare system is one of the world's premier systems because there is no rationing, she thinks, for example, that people don't have to wait for a year to have their hip replacement surgery, and she doesn't have to pay anything for her asthma medication. Getting inside this student's head helps us understand that for this relatively healthy student who has been fully covered by her parents' generous health insurance plan, there likely has been no rationing, no waiting in line, no prohibitive co-pays. Only when we pose interest in this way can we begin to help the student understand the detailed misery and tragic daily experiences of the underinsured and uninsured in our healthcare system.

As another example, recently three senior students stopped in my office as they were preparing their evidence-based practice paper about hydration and urinary tract infections (UTIs) in long-term care. They were stuck in the outcomes section of their project. Although they had identified the UTI rates as benchmarks for an outcome, they also listed "check I & O every 8 hrs" and "daily weights" as additional outcomes. Remembering that two of the students, Jenna and Corey, were employed as CNAs in nursing homes and were familiar with that setting, staff, and population, I tried using that information to help them examine outcomes more intensely and practically.

"Jenna, you've just come in to work the night shift, you're one CNA short, and you're told that you need to do an I & O and a daily weight on all 14 residents by the end of your shift at 7 a.m."

Jenna groaned and griped, as she burst into a chuckle, "It would never happen!" Corey immediately assumed his role, "But this is for a *research* project . . . they're measuring hydration and UTIs."

We all laughed and the three students quickly identified the importance of feasibility, the real world in outcome measurement. Perhaps from a novice, academic, or textbook perspective, I & Os every 8 hours and daily weights on all residents in the nursing home were *reasonable* outcomes. But integrating the students' work experiences helped them understand the futility of these strategies. Getting inside the students' head to imagine their apprentice standpoint and also their out-of-class experiences can be central in posing interest.

Our teaching demands that we do this. Our teaching cannot be focused on what mistakes students make, what they don't understand. Even more distressing than emphasizing students' errors are the faculty comments about how unmotivated, lazy, and small-minded students are today compared to "when *I* was a student." These good ole days comments barricade us from really getting inside the students' heads; they only prolong our paying attention rather than posing interest.

In the same essay mentioned earlier, Dr. Shulman (2004) proclaimed that the *right analogy*, based on a wide body of research, is "perhaps the most powerful tool a teacher has" (p. 412). Taking this idea one step further, we will know it is the right analogy if we know what is inside the students' head. Taking yet another step to close the loop, we will know what is inside the students' head only if we pose interest.

I'm not at all practiced in using meaningful analogies; the parallels I select seem dated, shallow, even dry. I've tried to use a few analogies: (1) comparing cerebral edema to a swelling balloon in a covered pint glass jar, (2) describing the transition from student to beginning staff nurse as a trapeze artist high in the big-top letting go of one swing and not yet gripping the next swing, and (3) equating surgical repair of a hemorrhaging liver to sewing up a soaked sponge or cotton candy. There you see—I told you analogies are not my forte. Perhaps I need to ask the students to craft some *right analogies*—now that could be a useful activity to help me get inside the students' heads.

"A FRIEND OF YOUR MIND" AND NAMASTE

As we are reminded by Alice James lying on her "forever couch" in the 19th century, when we pose interest with students we do not merely attend to their predicaments. We unite with them and who they are. We pose interest to establish presence with students in both clinical and classroom teaching by showing up, circulating, and getting inside the students' heads.

In closing, I'd like to borrow again from the imagination of Dr. Greene (1995, p. 38) as she persuades us to teach with imagination, to imagine invisibility, to pose interest by imagining the other. She calls on one of the characters in Toni Morrison's *Beloved* to help us see imagination. The character describes how he felt about a woman: "She is a friend of my mind. She gather me, man. The pieces I am, she gather them and give them back to me all in the right order. It's good, you know, when you got a woman who is a friend of your mind."

Our challenge in posing interest, then, is to be friends of the students' minds. In that friendship, we gather the pieces, gift them back, and help create wholeness.

As we become friends of the students' minds, our posing interest can be elegantly summarized in the respectful Hindu greeting *Namaste* (pronounced *nah-mah-stay*). It is used both for saying hello and good-bye and is usually accompanied by a slight bow, with the palms pressed together at the chest and fingertips pointing upward. Common translations include "I bow to you," "I reverently salute you," "I acknowledge the divine presence in you." Am I the only one who is struck by the comparison of this greeting to the usual stunted, skeletal "Hi" and "Bye"?

In the spirit of friendship, teaching them all, showing up, circulating, and getting inside the students' head, I salute you: *Namaste.*

REFERENCES

Greene, M. (1995). *Releasing the imagination: Essays on education, the arts, and social change.* San Francisco: Jossey-Bass.

Oates, J. C. (2003). *The faith of a writer: Life, craft, art.* New York: HarperCollins.

Palmer, P. J. (2004). *A hidden wholeness: The journey toward an undivided life.* San Francisco: Jossey-Bass.

Phillips, D. T. (1992). *Lincoln on leadership: Executive strategies for tough times.* New York: Warner Books.

Shulman, L. S. (2004). *The wisdom of practice: Essays on teaching, learning, and learning to teach.* San Francisco: Jossey-Bass.

Thaler, R. H., & Sunstein, C. R. (2008). *Nudge: Improving decisions about health, wealth, and happiness.* New Haven, CT: Yale University Press.

Teaching Practices That I Am Practicing

CHAPTER 8

Clinical Teaching Is Where the Magic Lies

The erasure of a human subspecies is largely painless—to us—if we know little enough about it. . . . We grieve only for what we know. The erasure of Silphium from western Dane County is no cause for grief if one knows it only as a name in a botany book.

—Aldo Leopold

New nurse educators come to be in academic positions in a mix of ways. Phrases like "stumble upon," "flight from," "begged to," "dreamt for," or perhaps "blindly persuaded" describe the passageway. Stumbles or begs or dreams aside, often clinical teaching is the first landing as nurses assume faculty roles. Although this can be a rough and rutted arrival for the new teacher, clinical education is where students come to know nursing.

We don't care much about things we don't know. The roadside spaces and cemetery corners of Leopold's Sand County are where Silphium, that giant yellow native prairie flower, unfurls. We come to care about Silphium when we know it in those spaces and corners, far beyond a name in a botany book.

So, too, health and illness unfold in clinical education, far removed from the often barren and bony concepts discussed in textbooks. It is in that unfolding, it is in clinical education where we come to know nursing, where we come to care—and therein lies the magic.

A dean of nursing once told me that the most skilled and experienced educators should primarily be responsible for clinical teaching in any nursing program. Although this was not occurring in the program she administered, her point was that clinical education prickles with more knacks and intricacies than classroom teaching does. In this chapter, I highlight some of the challenges of clinical teaching and offer suggestions for a smoother landing for the new clinical educator.

CLINICAL EDUCATION AS THE PINNACLE OF COMPLEXITY

Jeffrey Kluger's (2008) Complexity Arc proffers an exquisite model for understanding clinical teaching. In this bell-shaped arc, the *complexity* is highest in the middle with *simplicity* falling at either end of the arc. Chaos and instability surface as one type of simplicity at one end of the arc; for example, this type of simplicity could be represented by light traffic with cars going every which way, any way they please. At the other end of the arc, in another type of simplicity, lies a static and robust state; this could be represented by traffic gridlock with cars going nearly nowhere. Kluger describes these two simplicity states as "spinning disorder at one end and flash frozen order at the other" (p. 28), neither of which is very complex.

At the top of the curve, however, lies the most complex spot on the arc. The most unsteadily and perilously poised situation is at the top. Continuing the traffic example, with traffic speeds ranging from 25 to 45 miles per hour and between 5000 and 6000 vehicles passing a given point each hour, nearly any tiny thing can tip the balance into either chaos or gridlock. The playmaker may be a distracted cell phone user, a mother driver tending to a crying infant, a traffic jam in another section of the city, or an extra busy on ramp—hence the complexity.

Admittedly, complexity is a shifty and dodgy idea. For example, things that we might consider complex, because of their enormous size, prolonged life span, soaring cost, or shimmering glitz, actually may be outrageously simple. The opposite is true as well; things that seem extraordinarily simple may be remarkably complex.

To make this point, Kluger (2008) proposes that a pencil perches at the top of the complexity arc. It is not huge, it doesn't cost much, it doesn't live very long, and it's not flashy—but it is complex. The pencil begins as a cedar sapling, a chunk of raw material in a bauxite mine, a lump of carbon in the coal belt, and a cooked rubber eraser in a lab. Further, this paltry pencil requires a vast number of supporting people and industries before it turns up in our hands, sharp and snappy. The short-lived guppy, which Kluger describes as a "symphony of systems" is another example of complexity.

The pencil and the guppy and certainly a human handshake out-complex a simple star that is merely a furnace "made up of three layers of gases that slam hydrogen atoms together into helium, release a little light and fire in the process, and achieve nothing more than that" (Kluger, 2008, p. 12). Yet we may be tempted to place that star at the top of the complexity arc because of its size, distance, and light, as well as the reverence we have always granted it.

Nonetheless, determining complexity is complex in itself. Assessments about complexity must be made both up close and at a distance. "Interesting" and "active" indicate complexity. "Hard," "lumpish," and "fixed" argue for simplicity. The more precarious the balance at the top of the arc, the more complex the situation. One way of deciding whether something is simple or complex, albeit a hurried and superficial approach, is by answering the question, "How hard is it to describe?"

Clinical education is unspeakably hard to describe. Up close and at a distance, it is exciting and certainly active. Clinical education hovers merely minutes from chaos and instability, on the one hand, and inches toward standstill on the other. The students who are not clear about their goals or who have a serious problem with disorganization illustrate the instability. Only minutes away, the students immobilized by anxiety, lack of knowledge, or a flighty and erratic staff preceptor reflect the standstill.

Just as the students may drift between instability and standstill, new clinical educators also can easily collapse into the chaos or the static ends of the complexity arc. As part of this wobbly balance, the clinical educator juggles numerous critical players in the educational process: (1) the client, (2) the client's family or other people of significance, (3) the student, (3) the registered nurse who has primary responsibility for the client in the clinical setting, and (4) other healthcare providers, including physicians, therapists, and social workers.

Moreover, the number of these key players is further multiplied. At any given time, the clinical educator is directly responsible for 8 or 10 students, and each of the students may be providing care for one to four clients. This all occurs within two distinct but intersecting systems simultaneously: the education system and the healthcare system. These two systems have very different purposes, philosophies, economic motives, organizational structures, languages, and computer systems. Finally, an individual clinical educator may be teaching different levels of students in more than one healthcare setting during the same semester. It goes without saying, there are specific educational outcomes based in the curriculum that all students are expected to achieve.

To sum the circumstances, then, there are multiple individual players within two very diverse but overlapping systems that are directed by divergent goals. These circumstances are frequently further complicated when the clinical educator is teaching students from various levels in the program in different healthcare settings. To top it off, the clinical instructor is new to the role. Nothing lumpish or fixed about any of this!

This portrayal highlights the "who" and perhaps hints at the "what" in the complexity of clinical education, but the "how" pleads for help. How can we keep clinical education at the top of the complexity arc? How can we prevent it from skidding back into the spinning disorder of chaos and instability, on the one hand, or flash-freezing into educational and emotional gridlock where individuals and the teaching–learning process are paralyzed? How can the clinical educator proceed within this complexity and be effective at the top of this complexity arc?

PREPARING FOR DEPARTURE

Three key strategies may help prepare for the clinical educator position. First, in addition to reviewing the course focus and objectives, clarifying and internalizing the specific clinical outcomes, skills, or competencies are essential. What are students expected to learn in their clinical experience? How has that been taught in the past? What specific types of patient or family assignments benefit the students? How are clinical outcomes evaluated? What is particularly challenging for the students in this course? A beginning clinical educator *must* ask course colleagues or an immediate supervisor these questions and have a solid understanding of the answers.

It is often blindly believed that a new clinical educator will "just know how to teach in clinical" because that individual is an expert nurse in clinical practice. Not only do other faculty frequently assume this, but novice educators also assume this about themselves. This presumption is rarely true—nursing practice is distinctly different from nursing education. Each has its own body of knowledge and each requires application of a unique research base. Being trapped in this assumption pulls you into a quagmire where you may be hesitant to ask questions, feel embarrassed about not knowing, overlook unsafe or unacceptable student practice, or mishandle delicate and complex student performance situations. Thus, being honest and clear about being a new clinical educator is essential. When clinical education is envisioned at the top of the complexity arc, the demand for honesty and clarity is unquestioned.

In addition to becoming immersed in the clinical course you are teaching, it is also helpful to briefly survey the concurrent nursing courses and experiences in which the students are enrolled. Review the other course syllabi and meet with the faculty teaching those courses to find out the overall goal of the course, major topic areas, and substantial assignments and due dates. In this way the clinical educator can "see" the semester texture from the students' perspective and perhaps interlock significant learning experiences. Particularly demanding times for students can also be anticipated.

A second strategy to prepare for the clinical educator position is to examine your own past experiences. That is, what clinical experiences have you had while you were a student that were particularly meaningful? I suggest delving into this detail as much as possible. One suggestion is to write about a past clinical experience or a course that you recall; this writing will expand your discovery. For example, you may remember an incident from your senior year when you had difficulty caring for a patient who was an alcoholic driving a car in an accident where a 24-year-old young father and his toddler daughter were killed. Try writing responses to a range of questions. What happened during that day in your clinical experience? What did the instructor do? What do you wish the instructor would have done? What did you (and perhaps other students) do before, during, and after the experience? What do you think now about this experience?

Besides examining your own student clinical learning, it may be beneficial to recall the experiences you may have had as a staff nurse or in a managerial position. It is likely that you were able to observe other clinical instructors teaching and learning with students from a nearby nursing program. For instance, you may have seen an instructor work with a student who made a medication error or could not draw linkages between lab results and pathophysiology. From your staff nurse perspective, what did you see that was particularly meaningful for the students, the patients, the staff? How did the instructor pose questions? How did the students respond? Again, writing about several observations will help you recall and interpret the significance of them.

A third strategy to prepare for clinical teaching is absolutely essential: Orient yourself to the clinical setting. This may require several days of providing direct patient care with a staff nurse preceptor. The emphasis here is to review types of patients, their medications and treatments, and unit routines and documentation requirements, as well as to meet other healthcare providers. You can arrange an orientation with the first-line nurse manager or educator on the unit. In some healthcare systems, one individual has institution-wide responsibility for coordinating and scheduling student clinical experiences. More and more students and programs compete for days and times on units; this necessitates overall coordination and sometimes results in very limited opportunity for student placement.

Not only does an orientation help you review patient care, but it also helps you meet a variety of nursing staff. Without meaning to sound insensitive, it is important to identify which individuals are most willing, patient, and able to teach and learn with nursing students. Knowing this helps you make effective student assignments (especially for students who may be struggling in the clinical setting). In sticky situations, it also helps to know who is generally supportive of nursing education and professional development. Last, a clinical instructor's credibility with the unit staff is markedly enhanced if the staff see new educators taking direct steps to become oriented. Through these actions, the new clinical educator cultivates a more accommodating and forgiving environment.

Your preparation for the clinical teaching role must be deliberate and planned. It is simply too risky to assume that your clinical practice expertise will suffice as you and the students clutch the top of the complexity arc. Clearly, understanding clinical outcomes, examining past experiences, and orienting to the clinical unit are indispensable—know the course, know yourself, and know the clinical setting before you depart.

IN FLIGHT

After you have intentionally prepared for the clinical teaching position, what are strategies that will help you fly forward? Although germane to both clinical and classroom teaching, four areas are especially relevant to beginning as a clinical educator: (1) relationships with teaching colleagues, (2) relationships with students, (3) helping students learn to think, and (4) covering the content—less is more.

Relationships with Teaching Colleagues

Often, new clinical educators feel isolated in their role. Frequently, they hold part-time positions, with little or no classroom teaching responsibilities or other service or scholarly activities that bring them to campus. As a result, they feel little connection with other faculty in the nursing program and even less connection with other campus employees.

To help counteract this disengagement, forging relationships with nursing and nonnursing colleagues is needed. At a minimum, make every effort to participate in course meetings. Typically, there is a team of instructors involved in a single course, especially if there is a clinical component. This team usually has planned course meetings (often weekly or biweekly) to review course activities, clinical progress, student issues, and the like. Attending these meetings is vital. If you cannot attend face-to-face meetings, you may have the opportunity to use phone, audio, video, or other tech solutions to be present. Not only will your immersion in the course be strengthened, but the students' learning will be significantly enhanced because you will be more familiar with course objectives and learn from other course faculty.

This dialogue with other faculty results in all sorts of help. Relationships are established in which future, often tricky, issues can be discussed (e.g., a student's poor performance or how one manages when several patients refuse care from a student from a minority background or for whom English is a second language). Unwritten do's and don'ts are learned; that is, what are acceptable grade parameters for clinical written work, and how students' performance appraisals are written or their clinical files are handled. How-to's are shared. For example, there are grids or organizational charts that help track (1) students' experiences and their areas of strength and need, (2) types of patients, and (3) assignment due dates and submissions.

Bradley, a new clinical instructor, once admitted that he had expected to keep all of this student-specific information in his head. Because as a critical care staff nurse he was used to keeping lots of patient details at the tip of his fingers and he had a great memory, tracking only eight students seemed like it would be nearly mechanical. Needless to say, Bradley quickly learned to use a student grid to track this information because students, patients, experiences, and assignments began to mist and fog in his memory over the course of a 15-week semester. On one occasion, he needed to be absent from clinical for an unexpected family emergency, and unfortunately, there was no written record for the substituting clinical instructor. By using the grid, Bradley designed clinical experiences for each student more purposefully and more certainly. Because he did this, the students also became more direct in examining their own learning and what they still needed to accomplish. As a result, Bradley felt that he and the clinical group were not just putting in the hours; they were much more individually goal-directed.

Relationships with Students

As a new young clinical faculty, I remember my discomfort in being as old as or younger than (in some instances) the students in my clinical group. Usually, this was not an issue, but there were occasions when the age issue surfaced and I questioned my own skills, both as a nurse and as a teacher.

One approach that helped was to capitalize on the students' prior life experiences. For one student, this was her background as a veterinarian; for another it was his first profession as a mortician. Helping students link their previous experiences with nursing is key; for example, common patterns surface quickly between health care and a military tour of duty, parenting, or employment in retail or food service. So, instead of ignoring or minimizing them, I validate the students' experiences and, to the extent possible, entwine them with learning about nursing. Mingling life encounters in this way helps other students in the group examine their own past and culture and thereby augment their own learning; making connections also helps students develop a pattern-seeking sense of inquiry.

A word of caution: Take care not to glibly use a student's experience or identity (gender, race, age, religion, profession) as representative of a broader group. I recall one experience where I overemphasized one student's past experience; I finally saw the group's eye-rolling weariness when I continually incorporated the student's previous profession as a dietician. The group thought it stale and the dietician–student was also drained by it, I'm sure.

Helping Students Learn to Think

Although the idea of coaching may be a bit dated and sometimes criticized for being a sports analogy, there is some value in examining its underlying premises. At the start, the clinical teacher actually facilitates learning rather than gives information. The students must be active "performers," if you will, rather than you being the sole active performer while the students passively sit back like spectators. As a coach, then, your role may be to help students think and practice better as nurses. And it is that thinking and practice, over and over again, that are indispensable.

One way that I've learned to promote active learning and to help students reason, build, and think better is by thinking out loud with them. Thinking out loud lets the students *hear* you think, *see* you puzzle. Thinking out loud models the thinking we want students and liberally educated nurses to do.

In my early years of teaching, thinking out loud did not come naturally. Initially, an instant sparkly response to students' questions or clinical situations seemed essential. Anything less than a brainy glitter or an all-knowing shine felt unacceptable and far from professor-like. When I thought to myself in this way, the students did not see how I mulled over my thoughts and stumbled toward an answer because I did this silently and pondered mutely before imparting my glossy response.

The usefulness of the practice of thinking out loud is echoed in Paul and Elder's (2007) writing about critical thinking. They describe the need to model and call attention to specific "moves" in our thinking. One move, for example, is to *focus on implications.* In a nursing practice situation, the clinical instructor might say, "Whenever I'm thinking through a significant decision in patient care, I always try to think through the consequences or effects of what I do. What might happen if I withhold all analgesics for another hour? What might happen if I give the morphine now? What might happen if I give hydrocodone bitartrate and acetaminophen (Vicodin) instead of the morphine? What might happen if I use other interventions, such as repositioning or distraction or massage?"

A second move that Paul and Elder (2007) suggest is a *focus on clarity.* Responding to a student who describes an awkward or complicated incident with the staff RN and a patient's family, the clinical instructor might model this focus in the following way: "What you're describing seems like a complex situation. When I find myself in these kinds of difficult places, I really try to clarify the issue and details with all the people involved so that I am more clear about what happened. Talking with everyone helps me determine what I may be able to do. Please tell me all that you saw and heard, and then I will also discuss this incident with the staff RN and the patient's family."

A final move adapted from Paul and Elder (2007) is a *focus on intellectual honesty*. This is the thinking out loud associated with intellectual humility and intellectual courage. Through modeling, the students learn the "how" and "why" of admitting not knowing, as well as changing one's mind when additional information becomes available or when other, more reasonable arguments are heard. Students learn the value of critiquing their own thinking and behavior. Even though we may explicitly tell students that it's okay to make mistakes, unfortunately too often they are implicitly encouraged (by our nonverbal reactions or by receiving lower grades) to mask their thinking mistakes.

Thinking out loud with a focus on intellectual honesty, a clinical instructor might say, "I don't know what to do exactly, but I do know that . . ." or "I don't know for certain, but let's use the whiteboard to write down what we all know about this question, and then some ideas will emerge from our combined thoughts." Thus, knowledge is pooled, links are forged, and issues are broken down or put together in simpler terms that help all understand and remember.

Here's another example that models a focus on intellectual honesty: "Yesterday, when Jamie asked how to manage a certified nursing assistant whose performance was not acceptable, I responded with . . . But, when I thought about this further, I realized that my answer was superficial and did not take into account other considerations, like the organization's policy and procedure and nursing's Code of Ethics. I should have discussed all of these. This is a common problem in our thinking and dialogue: we go with our immediate response rather than taking enough time to consider more depth and viewpoints."

I would like to add another move of my own: a *focus on building*. Modeling this focus helps students learn to remember what they know and use that to construct new ideas or predict unfamiliar occurrences.

For example, in a clinical postconference, a student asks, "What happens to a patient with liver failure?" You freeze, recalling that it's been years since you've worked with an individual with liver dysfunction, and your knowledge of the lab tests and liver physiology blur into faraway murk. As you think out loud, however, you begin by listing what you and the students remember about normal liver function. Following a discussion of what the healthy liver does, the next step could be, "If these functions are affected (by alcohol abuse, infection, heart failure, or cancer), what might we see in the patient symptoms, lab tests, and treatments?" Again, you pool your knowledge and then build on it with a further question: "What other body systems would be changed and how?"

This focus on building helps students examine the familiar normal and then compare, observe, foresee what may be new to them. Of course, this is exactly the thinking that is essential in applying known principles to novel situations.

Covering the Content: Less Is More

Finally, as in classroom teaching, we must resist the temptation in clinical teaching to cover all the content. That is, we constantly must ask ourselves whether *we* are covering all the content or whether the *students* are covering the content. The instructor can give or cover large amounts of content in one course, but that is no guarantee that the students have internalized all that content, or made sense of it, or can begin to meaningfully apply it to problems or issues.

Sometimes faculty try to cover all the content in clinical experiences. They arrange for students to observe or be exposed to many different clinical settings, patients, procedures, units, and specialties—but, at the end of the day, little internalizing, practicing, or learning occurs for students. In all these settings, the students may merely observe passively while the staff nurse has largely been the doer, the practitioner, the thinker.

Lee Shulman (2004) addresses this trap of trying to cover all the content when he advocates that "less is more." He chides us not to be seduced by trying to cover everything, for that is easy, undemanding; in its place we must strive for the "depth, variation, and richness of the essential questions and central ideas of the disciplines" (p. 442).

It follows, then, that the challenge for us as clinical educators is to pinpoint the essential questions and central ideas of nursing in the clinical course we are teaching. Is it pain management? Is it safe medication administration? Is it helping patients and families live with chronic illness? Is it empowerment? Is it helping clients navigate the healthcare system? Is it helping families attend to aging parents? Is it having all students observe an obstetrical delivery? Is it having all students learn with a client from a culture different from their own? Is it complementary alternative therapies?

Shulman (2004) adamantly upholds that to focus on essential ideas, we don't simply decrease the amount of material to cover or we don't merely cover a shorter list of ideas more deeply. That is, we don't concentrate on nursing's essential ideas by trimming down a list of, for example, chronic pediatric pulmonary diseases from six to three and discussing those three in more depth. Instead, we may focus on family coping, health within illness, or ethical issues of justice or patient autonomy. "The ideas themselves change character . . . the more central a concept, principle, or skill to any discipline . . . the more likely it is to be irregular, ambiguous, elusive, puzzling, and resistant to simple . . . explanation. Thus, if we are to make less into more, we had better recognize that less is harder than more, less is more complex than more, less is more enigmatic or cryptic than more" (pp. 442, 443).

Perhaps it is just that—because less is more difficult, we shy away, shrinking back from uncovering the central essence of our discipline. We try to appease all educators, all settings, all specialty organizations, all possible turfs. Some of our program visions, missions, and frameworks read like the litany of all saints, or sometimes they are so nebulous they say little at all. Less is more insists that we clearly claim our core, individually and collectively.

CONCLUSION

Orienting to the course and the clinical setting as well as fully reflecting on student and staff nurse experiences prepare us to scale the complexity arc in clinical education. Day to day, as we cling to its top, our relationships with our teaching colleagues and the students provides a much-needed grip. The magic of our thinking moves charms and challenges us and also guards us from the instability and static ends of simplicity. And only when we can make less into more, when we can describe the "pencils," the "guppies," the "handshakes" of nursing as we teach and learn with students in clinical settings does nursing education emerge more richly as liberal education. And that is the pinnacle of complexity.

QUESTIONS TO PONDER

1. As you consider clinical education the Pinnacle of Complexity, what specific student-teacher experiences have you had in the clinical setting that illustrate this Pinnacle? What teaching approaches kept the situation from spinning into disorder or flashing into a freeze? Or, what factors pushed the situation from the top of the complexity pinnacle to one end or the other?

2. In evaluating students' performance in the clinical setting, it is unrealistic to assume that all students will be assessed without any teacher bias.

What biases may be most common for you? For your teaching colleagues? For healthcare agency staff? What are sources of this bias? How
can these biases be managed?

3. In the classroom content or the clinical setting that you teach, what are
"essential questions and central ideas?" What is the rationale for your
selection? In responding to this query, what questions need to be
answered first?

4. Perhaps clinical education is less glamorous and yet more complicated
than education in other settings. What justifications support this assumption? How might other groups of educators respond to this assumption?

REFERENCES

Kluger, J. (2008). *Simplexity: Why simple things become complex (and how complex things can
be made simple)*. New York: Hyperion.

Paul, R., & Elder, L. (2007). *A miniature guide for those who teach on how to improve student
learning: 30 practical ideas*. Dillon Beach, CA: Foundation for Critical Thinking Press.

Shulman, L. S. (2004). *The wisdom of practice: Essays on teaching, learning, and learning to
teach*. San Francisco: Jossey-Bass.

CHAPTER 9

The Novel: "Listen Her and She Will Show Us Everything"

When you only read things that you agree with, the mind becomes stagnant.

—Duane Alan Hahn

Specific facts consume our discipline. Particular descriptions and meticulous actions engulf our profession. As a result, students are learning-wedged in nursing's detailed swirl and gritty memorization. They lug around textbooks that exceed 10 pounds in weight, and their backs screech as their backpacks overflow. Each passing year stretches the length of textbook reading assignments.

Undeniably, textbooks matter, as do clinical experiences, writing activities, and other learning methods. But textbooks are usually formatted in a linear, repetitive, factually dense, often rigid framework. If textbooks are all the students read, might it be that as nurses they will think and talk like a textbook? And might they relate to their colleagues and clients like the textbook prescribes?

Clients, students, and colleagues tell us their lives in story form, not in textbook form. Thus, we need to make meaning from their *story*, their *humanity*.

Reading novels can help students discover meaning, connect patterns, and look for surprises in those stories. Mere memorization from the textbook will not achieve that envisioning. Beyond textbooks, novels must be part of a liberal nursing education and cannot be limited to a particular literature class.

The stories we hear—the humanity we try to understand—are the human responses that are the focus of our practice and the center of nursing education. We know that these responses are intricate and complex, often knotty, even thorny. That is, pain and suffering are complicated. Spiritual distress is fragile. Immobility may not be what it appears. Confusion can be feeble and yet sturdy at the same time. Relationships always come with a history. And yet, these complicated and delicate human stories are what we expect students to learn about, understand, and attend.

When nursing students learn about human responses and client decisions, they often maintain a simplistic understanding. Frequently, they cling to an appreciation of people and places like themselves, a perception sometimes bordering on absolutism. Reading a novel can unsettle those certainties. A novel can press us to unease, for when you read only things that you agree with, the mind becomes stagnant, as Duane Alan Hahn reminds us. A novel turns down the volume of our internal conversations, shakes us up, and makes us question our truths.

Still, that shakeup happens only when we deem the novel more than a symbol. Unless we experience the world of the novel, enter its life, and tremble and breathe with the characters and walk in their destiny, we will not be able to empathize. A novel pleads for empathy. It is in this empathy that we can more deeply understand human responses, which prevail at nursing's core.

LINKING NOVELS AND HUMAN RESPONSES

How people connect with each other is part of their human response. Reading a novel helps us appreciate connections, how they rise and grow, how they crack and collapse. In Pamela Gien's *The Syringa Tree* (2006), set in South Africa under apartheid in the 1960s, connections accelerate in iron friendships and also collide in steely jaws. The Afrikaans whispered about Lizzie Grace's physician father as "Jood," and "more disgusting even than that," about his wife who was "Katoliek." In Dr. Grace's office, the blacks' exam rooms were separated from the whites'; blacks edged up the back stairs to their section and whites walked up the front, heedless of their advantaged place. Lizzie described the majority of her father's patients as "Afrikaans, some English like us, a whole lot black, and a few in between." Lizzie's greatest love is Salamina, her Xhosa African tribal nanny. It is Salamina's newborn infant whom Lizzie illegally protects in the safe walls of her own home, at least safe for now.

Human connections collided with and splintered those walls. Loeska, the blue-eyed Afrikaans girl living across the bush-fence from Lizzie, announced that Lizzie "had grown into a stick insect with 'poo-tainted' eyes . . . *that's* why miggies [small bugs with wings] fly into them—drawn to cesspools." Loeska hatefully hammered those splinters even further as she screamed at Lizzie: it must be that you have "some *Jewish* in you or maybe even some *black*."

Experiencing these connections, as they are affected by race, gender, and class in *The Syringa Tree*, helps nursing students understand systems of privilege and oppression in society. A liberally educated nurse must examine these structures of difference. After recognizing how economic and sociological factors influence privilege and oppression, students begin to grasp, in turn, how the lives of individuals and groups are shaped. As a result, a clearer and more truthful insight about human responses emerges. In addition, not only can students begin to untangle their own position in these unequal power systems, but they can also dissect their personal perspective about others' position as well.

Reading a novel also helps us strip away the surface that meets the eye and curiously explore what is underneath. Reading a novel helps us ask questions. Norah, the 20-year-old daughter in Carol Shield's *Unless* (2002), slept in the Promise Hostel and spent her days sitting cross-legged on a square of street gripping a begging bowl in her lap. She scrawled "GOODNESS" across a flimsy cardboard sign and dangled it from her neck. What drove Norah out of her boyfriend's apartment and pushed her out of classes at the university? What was the scabby infection partially hidden by a string that gathered her shabby mitten to her tattered sleeve hem? How might Norah's powerlessness as a woman and current political activism have shackled her to that Toronto street corner?

Unless we ask these questions about Norah, we will never learn about her efforts at saving a Muslim woman who lit herself on fire in the middle of the street to protest her social and political situation. Unless we ask these questions, we will never learn about Norah's flight from the ER, her own burn injuries, her statement about "goodness," her posttraumatic human response. Through meeting Norah and entering her life, students also learn about the science and art of questioning clients, learn to grapple with the complexity of their lives, to see and hear their human responses.

So, reading a novel cultivates a new way of looking. Studying the connections and systems Lizzie confronted in South Africa and analyzing the life that dropped Norah on a Toronto square of pavement help us hold the intensity and embrace with empathy the many layers of human responses.

We rarely read a novel simply to ascertain whether the characters are good or bad, right or wrong, likeable or distasteful. We might be tempted to dismiss Loeska as a brat if we don't examine the societal systems of power inequality in which she lived or the evolution and consequences of her family's values. Or we might brush off Norah as a naïve ex-college student bent on social activism if we don't gently and deliberately pursue what is in hiding beneath this prejudgment. In novel reading, there is no place for lecturing, scolding, ranting.

As Nafisi (2003) reminds her Iranian students studying literature in *Reading Lolita in Tehran*, a good novel prevents us "from the self-righteousness that sees morality in fixed formulas about good and evil" (p. 133) and "creates enough space for all these characters to have a voice . . . not seeing [their problems and pains] means denying their existence" (p. 132). Nafisi further cautions the students, "Don't go chasing after the grand theme, the idea . . . as if it is separate from the story itself. The idea or ideas behind the story must come to you through the experience of the novel and not as something tacked on to it" (p. 109). For me, Nafisi is positioning the novel and its characters in the center, and as readers, we come to it plainly and gently, taking it in and going out to it.

REPOSITIONING NOVEL READING IN NURSING EDUCATION

How do nursing students learn to create enough spaces that grant voice to all clients? This question prompts us further: How do students learn about both the command of advantage and the vulnerability of disadvantage? Amy Tan (2005) explores these concepts in a Myanmar (Burmese) military and political setting in *Saving Fish from Drowning*. Sight, as both advantage and disadvantage, is powerfully portrayed in Nobel laureate José Saramago's (2008) *Blindness*. In a similar way, Ursula Hegi (1995) depicts dwarfism in *Stones from the River*.

And further: How do students discover systems? That is, how do they learn to look farther and farther upstream and long beyond the horizon? Kim Edwards (2006) in *The Memory Keeper's Daughter*, John Berendt (1999) in *Midnight in the Garden of Good and Evil* (nonfiction novel), Michael Dorris (2003) in *A Yellow Raft in Blue Water*, and Cormac McCarthy (2008) in *The Road* all can help students uncover the depth and breadth of family and community systems.

And even further: How can students really understand prevention? For example, how can students come to realize that it is not only volunteering at the food pantry that is essential but that ever more critical is helping to form a society in which there is no need for a food pantry? Unraveling the complexities of the rapidly expanding food handout programs in the United States may help students see poverty as hunger's root cause. A focus on prevention requires us to disentangle the following dimensions: (1) communities revved up to "put a turkey in every pot" at Thanksgiving, (2) swelling food distribution infrastructure demonstrated by growing lines at food kitchens and food stamp offices, (3) immediate gratification for both the donors and recipients, (4) role of the food industry viewing food banks as a waste-management tool, (5) political platforms, economic trends, and social class descriptions, as well as (6) a dependence on volunteers driven by the belief that they are helping by "feeding the hungry," perhaps affirmed by our campus service learning efforts.

Novels that plead with the reader to explore prevention are widespread. For example, novels about abuse, such as *Spencerville* by Nelson DeMille, *Black and Blue* by Anna Quindlen, and *Lovely Bones* by Alice Sebold, beg us to consider prevention, an essential but often abandoned, ill-funded, and unglamorous aspect of nursing and health care. Learning all of these lessons is our only hope for survival, and novel reading can help fulfill that vision.

NOVEL READING: BEYOND "BUSYWORK" AND "BORING"

Over the years, I have learned some techniques for integrating novel-reading into nursing education that have worked for the nursing students and for me. As always, in the beginning I tried some strategies that turned out to be virtually useless—where students protested novel reading as busywork, not related to nursing, boring, where typical student responses were "I got by without ever reading a word of it" and "lose it." But I wasn't ready to give up. Not only is reading novels one of my passions, but I am sure that novels can contribute to nursing education. I was certain that students could also be convinced of the value of novels.

In bringing novel reading to nursing education, selecting the novel is an important initial consideration. For me, asking the students to read a novel of their choice and then write a report about it, with no discussion in class, has been practically fruitless. Even when I've given students a choice from a precompiled list of titles, the results have been mixed. In those instances, I've been able to draw comparisons between novels in class discussion. Although this exercise stirs my own thinking, because I've read all the novels on the list, the students who have not read the titles mentioned are marginalized because they have not entered the life of the novel, breathed and trembled with its characters.

I have had more success by carefully selecting a novel for the entire class to read. To help me make a selection, sometimes I've asked the students to write down the titles of their two favorite books. This list helps me to see what they have read already and directs my selection. (Because Harry Potter is always right at the top of students' lists, I must think more about Harry's and Hermione's and Dumbledore's and Voldemort's human responses.) At any rate, when everyone reads the same novel, everyone is more engaged in discussion because there is less time to "text in or tune out," until "she gets to the one I read."

When I've discussed novel reading with faculty colleagues, invariably they will ask, "What is the best novel you can recommend?" I have no best novel because the characters in all novels live human responses that necessitate empathy. I use a shorter, rather than a longer novel and one I've read recently; it also helps if I've discussed the book with others because then I've entered into more of its life. I vary novels semester to semester and stay with contemporary works because I am most familiar with them.

In addition to selecting the novel, the teacher must help students hear and internalize the significant contribution novel reading can make to their learning about nursing. First, spending planned time in class describing the "why" of this learning activity is central. For example, highlight specific novels and how they can help us understand relationships among and between individuals and groups; learn to ask questions; examine sociological, economic, and family systems; and study topics such as prevention, leadership, and autonomy. Devoting class time affirms the assignment's importance. Neglecting this discussion altogether, or yelping brief comments as students are packing their bags, turning on their cell phones, and walking out the door signals busywork, a curricular snub if you will.

If course requirements are weighted by percentage or points, the novel-reading activities cannot be a lightweight. Designating only a few points or a minimal percentage is the hidden curriculum that tells students that this isn't valuable, it's only filling up space, it's not nearly as important as the exams, and it's only included so that the instructor can be creative.

After selecting the novel and establishing the learning value with the students, guide them in the novel-reading activity. I've learned that posing dull questions for them to address after reading the novel produces dull responses. Students write what is expected of them. Admittedly, I have used too many of these dreary queries myself: (1) describe the plot of the novel, (2) what human response(s) did you see in the novel? (3) who was your favorite character and why? and (4) in what way was the ending of the novel unexpected or expected for you? With these types of questions, the students morph most of the answers from the book flap or title, introduction or review, savvy conversation with friends, or Internet sources.

Rather than supplying a list of questions, I've discovered that combining a (1) substantial written paper (e.g., reaction paper) and (2) class discussion has greater merit. I ask students to react to the book (individually or in pairs) in the paper, rather than letting the *book itself write the paper* (Wheeler, 1979, p. 167). I emphasize the value of the class discussion, and frequently there are students asking for it; it is as if they want to hear others' perspectives—their classmates' and my own. By using the reaction paper and subsequent discussion, the challenge for me has been to lead the students to examine what they don't realize they know.

To uncover this realization I suggest the students create a dialogue between themselves and the novel. The emphasis is on their *experience with the novel*, not an *appreciation of it.* I ask the students to consider themselves as one circle, think about the novel as a second circle, and then bring the circles together so that they overlap. That overlap, the point or place where the circles meet or intersect most deeply, is what will mold the paper—it's not all novel and it's not all student. I advise them to actually draw two large overlapping circles before they begin reading and write thoughts about themselves in the first circle, striking points from the novel in the second circle, and their initial interpretations in the overlap. Sharing the circles in small groups partway through the novel reading helps them stay on track and results in richer detail.

By using this approach, the students write beyond themselves, beyond the novel. They write about ideas they discover in the overlap, and it is this discovery that shapes their thesis and also who they are as individuals. (Please see Figure 9-1 for an example.)

Discussing the focus of the reaction paper and providing some highlights in writing enriches the quality of the students' work. Again, spending some class time in this discussion underscores the value of novel reading. The goal of the reaction paper is to use the novel to rouse and stir ideas for both the students and the "readers." Each thesis and paper will be unique. Provide an example or two of a well-developed reaction paper online (for a novel different from the one the students are reading) to help allay student anxiety and carry their scholarship to a higher level. I encourage students to read the sample paper early in their novel reading and to begin asking the questions and exploring what lies underneath.

A simple, one-page handout about how to write the paper bolsters students' thinking and results in a stronger final product. This in-hand reference includes key ideas, with illustrating examples: (1) develop a bold, clear, interesting, and "gutsy" thesis that emerges from the circle overlap, (2) write to persuade the reader, not only to clarify for your self, (3) refrain from summarizing the plot (which describes and does not have a thesis or include your point of view), (4) use plot details to demonstrate a point—the details are a means to an end, not an end itself, and (5) think "how" and "why" to interpret the novel, not to outline it.

As the novel-reading activity continues to unfold, and to keep things moving forward, guided by students' concerns I routinely e-mail clarifications and suggestions to the entire class. After the papers are written, I use the thesis statements the students created to shape the in-class discussion. Often, the discussion begins in small groups and then the full class comes together.

Let's review where we've been in this novel-reading discussion. As the core of nursing, human responses are complex and delicate; involve individuals, families, and communities; and must be studied with diverse approaches. Novel reading invites us to learn about these responses and about ourselves in

---

Figure 9-1   A Student's Experience with *Middlesex* by Jeffrey Eugenides (2002)

Student's Circle:
- 21-year-old woman
- Major in nursing
- Irish-American ethnic background; first-generation college student
- Rural, upper Midwest, Catholic background
- Third of five living children; mother is in remission with breast cancer; one brother committed suicide
- Traveled out of the state once with aunt/uncle to Florida
- Employed currently in campus library; various jobs in high school
- Others describe me as hard-working, serious, quiet, kind, smart, a skilled athlete

Novel's Circle:
- "Ford English School Melting Pot" in Detroit; "melting" traditionally dressed immigrants in huge cauldron on stage and then all emerge in blue/gray suits, waving U.S. flag, to the tune of *Yankee Doodle*
- "Cutting in half" used symbolically: geopolitically (e.g., Cyprus, Berlin, Korea); personally (Callie as a hermaphrodite)
- Power of language: black/white relationships in Detroit in 1960s where uprising was termed a "Riot," not a "Revolution." Dictionary reader referred to synonyms at "monster" under the word "hermaphrodite."
- Several incidents of someone lying: (1) to get a passport to come to United States, (2) brother and sister falsifying romance on ship, later were married and became parents, (3) Callie making up identity and role after she fled New York City and physician/surgery there

Overlapping Circle:
- How has the identity of my immigrant ancestors been forcibly altered since they came to the United States? To what extent were they eager or reluctant to leave their Irish culture to be "American"?
- Is there always some "division" in who we are or in what things are? That is, might there always be an inside and an outside? Might there be what I see and what I don't see about other people or other things or events?
- How am I (and others) influenced by the use of specific terms or phrases? How should I select words to use?
- Age-old question of whether lying is acceptable in certain situations.

Thesis:
Although my culture is uniquely who I am and how I live, I must examine more deeply my culture's intricacy and depth, its light and its shadow-side, as well as the forces that can or already have altered or eroded it.

distinct and sustaining ways and, as a result, augments the quality of our nursing care and enlarges who we are as liberally educated people. This chapter offers some pedagogical considerations about novel reading in nursing education, but as with any pedagogical activity, nurse educators must continually sculpt and form it to fit for themselves, the students, and the context. This carving is shaped by who we are as teachers and championed by the learning that is ongoing for us and the students.

"LISTEN HER AND SHE WILL SHOW US EVERYTHING"

Please allow me to indulge in one final story—from a novel, naturally. This story illustrates the delicacy of listening, which may be one of the greatest acts of empathy. Listening not only grounds a nurse's understanding of human responses but also underpins the teacher–student educational experience.

As a historical novelist, Richard Slotkin (2000) persuasively re-created the life Abraham Lincoln might have lived in his Kentucky and Indiana youth. In an anecdote from Lincoln's childhood, Slotkin exposes the intricacies of listening. As a 10-year-old, Abe met Old Konkapot, an Indian who squatted near the Lincoln cabin, wore his lank hair long, and always knew when Abe was coming to visit.

The boy wanted to learn how to hunt: "I ain't no hunter, never shot at nothin' bigger'n squ'rl, and never hit one yet." Old Konkapot flashed his teeth-gone grin, sat a long time, mild and friendly, so quiet it seemed he wasn't even breathing, and finally whispered, "I show you listen. I show you hunt. . . . The skin of the earth was a thin dress laid on riches and powers. Listen her and she lifts her dress, she shows you—everything."

Abe realized that listening was Konkapot's hunting secret. Several days later, he returned to Konkapot's fire and patiently waited for more of the old Indian's whispers. Finally, Konkapot sighed gently, "If you wanted the good of critters, you had to learn to listen how they think, what makes them scared, when are they hungry and what do they like to eat and where would they look first to get it . . . men and critters got the same breath . . . get old, get shot— they die, both the same. Listen."

In his inquisitive wisdom, the child Lincoln asked his old friend, "How can a man know what a *critter* thinks? A *man* can't even tell what another *man* is thinking." And therein lies the delicacy of listening. Although the astute Konkapot understood the boy's challenge, he did not buy his assertion and tenderly "brushed the words off like dust."

Lincoln learned about listening at Konkapot's fire. So, too, the novel helps us understand the fragile complexity of human responses and clients' decisions. Only with that knowing can we engage in genuine dialogue and full discourse about ideas, issues, and choices—with the students and with our clients. The novel, then—we must "listen her, she will show us everything."

QUESTIONS TO PONDER

1. Discuss the assumptions that underlie using novel reading in nursing education. Do these assumptions always hold true? Why or why not?
2. Select a key essential question or central idea in the content that you teach. Propose a novel or nonfiction book that could be used to help students learn more about its ambiguity and its mystery. A librarian or book-reading friend may be helpful.
3. The overlapping circles is a framework that can be easily applied to facilitate students' understanding of complex issues. Similar to a concept map, what other ways can you apply this framework?
4. After identifying guidelines for a reaction paper that fits for you and your teaching, create a detailed rubric that can be shared with students and used in your evaluation of the paper. In using a rubric, what implications are there for the students and the educator?

REFERENCES

Eugenides, J. (2002). *Middlesex*. New York: Picador.

Gien, P. (2006). *The syringa tree*. New York: Random House.

Nafisi, A. (2003). *Reading Lolita in Tehran: A memoir in books*. New York: Random House.

Shields, C. (2002). *Unless*. New York: HarperCollins Publishers.

Slotkin, R. (2000). *Abe: A novel of the young Lincoln*. New York: Henry Holt and Company.

Wheeler, T. C. (1979). *The great American writing block: Causes and cures of the new illiteracy*. Middlesex, England: Penguin Books.

CHAPTER 10

The Students Co-Construct the Classroom

It is important that students bring a certain ragamuffin, barefoot irreverence to their studies; they are not here to worship what is known, but to question it.

—Jacob Bronowski

Students' ragamuffin and barefoot style may weld the new educator to the podium, rarely to step away or glance up. Picturing the students as irreverent—even cheeky and bold—may further solder teachers to their script and notes. Students' erratic and flippant questions may even threaten to send the new educator away trembling.

Yet, it was Jacob Bronowski, the mathematician–biologist whose Polish-Jewish family perished at Auschwitz, who condemned the dogma and ignorance of absolute knowledge, who warned that we must all think it possible that we may be mistaken. It was Dr. Bronowski who implored students to question what is known. Extending his directive even further, students must demand a voice in their learning and claim a space in our teaching, and with that determination, we are obligated to co-construct the classroom.

As a new educator, I frequently sidestepped students in my teaching and learning with them. Even now I sometimes evade students in my haste and thoughtlessness, or merely go through the motion of inclusion. This doesn't happen by design, of course. In fact, if asked about their role, I would unleash a zesty monologue about the essence of students' ideas, comments, and questions in creating a vivid classroom experience.

Admittedly, I do not bypass students intentionally, but it can result in a flimsy approach to inviting, affirming, and expanding their findings and our discovery. In this chapter, I highlight several practices that can help us—to help students—so that they can help us—co-construct the classroom. It is in this circular classroom space that we and the students can question what is known and engage together in teaching and learning.

SIMILAR EXPERIENCES, BUT WHAT MAKES THEM DIFFERENT?

I recently had one of these thin and shabby experiences in which I seemed to bypass students. In that experience, I had asked graduate students to prepare for class by reading two chapters about gender and diversity in leadership. To facilitate the discussion and encourage everyone's voice in the dialogue, I divided the class of 34 students into groups of 5 or 6 and invited them to respond to several questions: What did you learn? What questions would you ask the authors? What link can you make between the chapters and your own practice settings? What was the most unusual thing you read?

As the groups talked, the room was filled with energy and a growing force around ideas. As I weaved around the groups, I could hear well-developed viewpoints, insightful questions, and a strong beginning application to students' own leadership experience.

After 20 minutes, we came back together as a class and I asked for group responses. Two groups replied with a cursory, two-sentence summary of their discussion. I asked for more comments, but there was just blank and gap. What happened to all of the spirit I heard only minutes before? Was everyone really "all talked out"? Thinking I had not prepared well for the class and that I wasn't asking the right questions, we moved on to swiftly tidy up the ragged ends of the discussion. Probably we all felt a bit uneasy, feeble, and gloomy. I asked myself, "What just happened here?" Am I really that dry, dull, and preachy?

I've frequently seen this "re-tiring re-coil" phenomenon develop in this way. Initially there is dynamic small group discussion, but when the groups are reporting back, others seem to zone out. It is as if people are saying, "I've had my say and my listen in the small group, now I'm finished and I'm really not interested in hearing the monotonous reports from all the other groups. I don't think there will be anything new or different from what our group already said. Besides, I must think about my patient assignment for tomorrow morning, plan for the kid's dentist appointment after school, and catch up with my planner."

On the other hand, I have had successful small group/large group experiences as well. I recall other similar classes that evolved into full large-group dialogue that grew deeper, more concentrated and meaningful, and more and more inclusive. What did I do differently in those other situations? Both classes began in the same way: small groups to discuss three or four posed questions, and then an entire class regroup.

There were some differences. When the result was a lively and inclusive large-group discussion, during the small group discussion, I had circulated among the groups, sat at the tables with the students, and expanded, clarified, and questioned with them. Briefly joining some of the small groups helped me move comfortably around the room, made it easier to invite, listen, and affirm, and provided me with the details for subsequent small group reports. These details often are not reported to the large group and yet may be the meatiest, most delicate, or "lived" discussion. If I've heard the details, I can use them to add a humorous twist or drive a point home during the group reports.

In these richer learning experiences, when the small groups came back together, I divided the whiteboard into three columns, heading each with a summary phrase from the three questions (i.e., key point, application to practice, and question for the author). By calling a student's name from each of the groups, I deliberately requested a response to every question from all of the groups. As the students responded, I wrote a synopsis of their comment in the appropriate column. As part of this expected small group report, I affirmed students' ideas by using their names and visually presenting their thoughts in writing to the entire class.

Further, as I heard the student's comments, I would ask for clarification: "Leslie, if I summarize this as 'women's frequent use of avoidance in managing conflict,' would that accurately reflect your group's conclusion?" In this way, the students heard their name, heard the key point twice (from the student and from me), and saw it written on the board. At this time I could also add some details, dilemmas, or perspectives that I heard in the small group discussion when I participated at their table—again, to affirm and enrich.

In addition to emphasizing the key point in several ways, I also modeled *accountable talk*. This is done by asking the next small group, "Janet, how did your group's discussion about women's approach to conflict compare to Leslie's group's?" Accountable talk can also effectively highlight students' experiences: "Shannon described an extremely unfortunate incident around diversity that he had with a nurse manager. Did any other group discuss similar incidents of prejudice or perhaps an opposite experience where diversity was honored?"

With accountable talk, students are encouraged to describe their opinion or perspective, or convey an idea from the literature, in relation to the previous speaker. Consequently, a more connected dialogue is created. In some situations, I have explicitly asked students to tie their comments with those of an earlier speaker or pose a question to that individual. Accountable talk helps all of us move away from being an isolated learner and closer to being a part of a collaborative network of scholars.

As the students made the points in the three columns, they constructed the classroom experience. In my response to the students, I linked their comments to other literature about the topic, existing research, and my own experiences, most of which I had in my lecture notes. With classroom co-construction, my goal is that no student will be a "full-time nobody."

RELENTLESS PREPARATION

Preparing for this type of student classroom construction is extensive and requires self-confidence, risk taking, and centeredness as an educator. I am reminded here of Rudolph Giuliani's (2002) demand for "relentless prepara- tion" (pp. 52–61) in his work as the New York City mayor. He maintained that preparation was the key factor in his success and that it relied on his ability to "visualize things in your own mind . . . learning something so thoroughly that it was part of my history."

Relentless preparation is time-intensive and likely not possible for every class the first time you teach it. Part of my ongoing preparation is learning all of the students' names (including correct pronunciations and nicknames, if I feel comfortable using them) and getting to know students individually as quickly as possible. Class pictures help, as do brief before and after class con- versations about, for example, their swim team accomplishments, daughter's concert, nursing assistant employment, or recent Hurricane Katrina volunteer experiences.

At the risk of overstating, I would like to emphasize that learning and using students' names are priceless practices. I seek to use names frequently, in and outside the classroom, verbally and in writing. I do all I can to consistently learn them, although this skill is tarnishing a bit as the years carry on and I find myself asking more often, "Can you please tell me your name once again?" But I have promised myself never to stop asking.

The "story of your name" is also a strategy that can help make students' names stick for me and facilitate classroom introductions (Lepp & Zorn, 2002, p. 385). Using various approaches, depending on the situation (e.g., in pairs, small groups, or in the larger class), students are asked to discuss the story of their name. After silently reflecting for 3 or 4 minutes on several of the fol- lowing questions, the students describe their name by sharing their responses orally: (1) How was your name selected? (2) Were you named after someone else, such as a relative, elder, movie star? (3) What meaning does your name have in another culture or language? (4) Do you have a different name in certain settings, such as at work, at play, with friends, at school, or with your family? and (5) Have you changed your name or has your family name been changed in the past?

I've learned some poignant, sometimes painful name stories. Elizabeth was named after her father's first love (who was not her mother). Jordan changed her name when she was 12 years old after discovering that she was named after an older sister who had survived only 2 weeks of life—"I hated seeing my name on the tombstone in the cemetery, so I picked a new name." I also learned that May Brooks feels terribly guilty for assuming her husband's last name rather than keeping her family name and remaining May Yang after she married. Also, Aaron Aadelot tells us that his father wanted a name for him that would always be at the very front of the alphabet. Sondra has totally given up when others call her Sandra. And as a teenager, Harriet abhorred her name but now she believes it is "just so classy."

In the story of your name activity, individuals are introduced based on *who* they are rather than on *what* they do or *where* they live. When I've used this strategy, I've discovered that the playing field levels, the energy level in the room skyrockets (after a moment of warm-up, people typically find it irresistible), and, from the stories I hear, remembering the students' names becomes nearly effortless thereafter.

In thinking about students' names, I'm reminded about the crushing experience that Eva Hoffman describes in *Lost in Translation* (1989). As children, Eva and her sister Alina's Polish names were bastardized upon their immigration to the western Canadian, English-speaking classes. Eva stalwartly reminds us that "our Polish names didn't *refer* to us; they *were* us as our eyes or hands [emphasis added]. . . . These new appellations . . . are not us. They are identification tags . . . names that make us strangers to ourselves" (p. 105). I resolve once again to inquire about correct name pronunciation, practice that pronunciation, and ask for help as often as I need it.

Relentless preparation means getting to know the students and their names, but it also means grooming the content. To plan for each class meeting, I identify key points about the topic and detail them sufficiently in writing, using an outline format rather than a full sentence narrative. Although I have seen some new educators write out their lecture word for word, I have found that writing complete sentences and paragraphs encourages me to read my notes and makes it more difficult to spot major ideas. As a result, I am more tethered to my notes, rather than joined with the students.

Instead, in addition to the key points in an outline, I write only a few bulleted items. This bulleted list includes a few descriptors about a study or two, as well as a phrase that reminds me of a hypothetical anecdote or a personal experience that I can use to supplement the students' classroom construction. I've also jotted down ahead of time several critical thinking questions so that I don't need to create these on the spot. My notes are very openly spaced, in large print, and well highlighted. I am very familiar with what I have written (nearly committing the major points to memory).

A student once told me that "it seems like you know this content so well, that you're able to 'play with it' when you teach." I treasured the comment deeply, but realize that it isn't always like this—undoubtedly not the first time I teach a class. But the playfulness became a vision for me. Play seemed an ideal metaphor that reflected liveliness, radiated good humor, and required partners or mates. Although we may label it *collaboration*, it is students co-constructing the classroom, nonetheless.

TAKE A BREAK

Throughout the class session, purposeful pauses are essential to maintain and strengthen the focus. These pauses are akin to grouping ideas into paragraphs in writing or scheduling spring breaks in the academic semester. As a novice educator, I did not appreciate the value of taking a deep breath—actually, I concentrated on sustaining nonstop "speak" so that any silence whatsoever would be prevented.

Now, not only do I give myself the freedom to consult my notes in class as needed, I've learned that a pause is essential for me. I take a break; sometimes I say, "Let me check my notes to see if there is anything else I would like to add to this idea." This pause helps me reflect momentarily and also provides some silence for thinking in the classroom. I have found that if I am comfortable with silence, the students become comfortable as well.

In addition, often close to the end of class, I pause and invite the students to review their notes, encouraging their questions for clarification or need for further discussion. Again, the reassuring calm of silence is critical for this consideration. Sometimes this closure activity generates topics for the next class—in this way, the students continue the classroom construction.

STUDENTS AND COURSE ASSIGNMENTS CO-CONSTRUCT THE CLASSROOM

When students begin to develop an idea or topic area for a paper or project, this early work can become a highly valuable component of classroom co-construction. For example, a course assignment may require that students (1) pose a barebones research question to guide a literature review summary or (2) choose a topic area for a paper. These questions or topic areas can be used as "live examples" to help the entire class move their thinking and writing forward.

A specific illustration may be helpful here. After choosing a topic for her literature review paper, Allison willingly shares her guiding question with the class: "Do herbal remedies cure colds?" With a bit of a coax, she writes her question on the whiteboard (or under the document camera) so that it is visible to everyone. Naturally, this requires her to move about the room and changes the room's character from "teacher standing in front being the only one speaking while all students listen" to a more open dialogue among teacher and students.

Several questions help affirm Allison as a curious learner and the value of her topic. In addition, other comments may help her narrow and specify her paper's question to make it more manageable and to help her move forward in developing the paper.

First, a question about *background* offers a solid place to begin. As Allison finishes writing her question on the whiteboard, I ask, "Can you tell us, please, what sparked your interest in this topic?" She describes her family's wide use of a variety of herbal remedies for the common cold and the fact that she has always questioned their effectiveness. A few follow-up questions asking for more detail might be useful here, such as, Can you give us some examples? What was the most frequent herbal used? How did your family accept or not accept these approaches? As a result, Allison speaks and the other students and I listen and learn.

Second, I might continue with a strong *affirmation* of the importance of her topic, noting the general increased use of herbal supplements and increased number of questions about them from clients. Asking for a show of hands, I probe the class, "How many in the room use some sort of herbal supplements?" The class hands and my own also avow the value of Allison's topic.

Third, other questions and observations may help *tighten and detail* everyone's guiding questions for their literature review paper. Here, it may be extremely beneficial to remind students of the need to restrict their paper topic because students often try to cover much too broad an area: "As you continue to develop your paper, you need to narrow and deepen the focus. This probably applies to many in the class. I suspect your topics begin as broad areas—but writing about too large an issue results in only a superficial, thin look at the topic. The goal in this paper is to taper your topic so that your examination of it becomes deeper and more detailed. This depth and detail moves your paper from a beginning college level to junior/senior level work."

Using Allison's topic can help demonstrate this direction for the class. "Allison, you identified Echinacea as one of the most commonly used herbs in your family. To help narrow and deepen the focus of your paper so that you're not trying to cover all the herbal remedies, it may work to select Echinacea or one of the other herbs used in your family as the topic. If you choose Echinacea, another way to limit your topic may be to examine the research about this herb as prevention versus a treatment for symptoms of the common cold."

Helping students tighten and detail their work is needed frequently. I've learned other guidelines that may help students focus their work: (1) limit the topic to a certain age group, such as school-age children, teens, middle-age or older adults, (2) focus on a specific area of practice, such as public health or acute care, or (3) restrict research to a particular historical period. On the other hand, in some situations students may be too narrow in their focus and need suggestions to expand their topic to other countries, disciplines, age groups, practice areas, or cultures other than their own.

Finally, comments and questions help ensure that students *understand the major components of the paper*. A simple question may be useful: "Allison, what do you think is going to be the most challenging part of this paper for you?" What is challenging for Allison is also likely to be difficult for others. This creates an opportunity to review specific ways to help students strengthen those areas.

From your own experience with past papers where students have had difficulty, you may also add, "As you develop your paper further, you'll need to remember to provide a conclusion to your review of research. In that review or synthesis, try to highlight what is already known and what gaps still exist in the research. In the past, students have struggled with that piece."

Here, you could display a few sample sentences or distribute them as a handout for the class. Here is an example of this type of conclusion: "The research describes what physiological and emotional adjustments there are in the first three months after gastric bypass surgery, but this research has included largely Caucasian women. The long-term adjustments, such as those occurring in 12 to 24 months, have not been studied. Further, women and men from minority populations have not been represented. Also, most of the research has been descriptive and no research could be found in which nursing interventions have been tested."

To review, this strategy of using course assignments to co-construct the classroom helps students and faculty actively engage in teaching and learning. Learning about the background of students and their topics, affirming their topic selection, helping them narrow and deepen their choices, and reviewing priority components of the assignment are approaches that offer a structure for this co-construction.

Introducing these approaches with an emphasis on learning, development, and collegial helpfulness, and not on evaluation or finding mistakes, is critical. Sometimes, depending on the class culture and topic, it may work to ask the class for their feedback (remember the need for adequate wait times). For example, "What suggestions do others have for Allison as she considers her paper topic?" Or, "I'm not familiar with this topic. What do others know about this?" In addition, following a discussion about one student's work, a way to move forward may be to invite others, "Is there anyone else who has a topic or approach that is very different from Allison's? Is there anyone who is really stumped about what to do or where to go?"

I must offer a few words of caution in using this co-construction strategy. First, this approach may be a little risky for the new educator because there is a need to think on your feet, an essence of spontaneity, and always a sense of the unknown, but I believe it can be effective just the same. If you find yourself in one of these "out of the blue" situations, there are always some saving graces, such as the following: (1) "I'm not sure exactly what to say, but the things I would think about are . . ." Or (2) "I've not seen this before. You're very creative. Can you tell us a bit more about what you're thinking here?" Or (3) "I need a little more time to think about this. Let's talk more after class."

The second caution is one that I've just been reminded of this past semester. A graduate student noted on her course evaluation that I spent nearly 1 hour on one student's research proposal while "this time could have been spent on my own proposal." Yikes! I intended for my dialogue with the individual student to be applicable to all or most students in the class, but apparently, it was not perceived in that way by everyone. This is a reminder for me not only to "keep it short" for an individual student, but also to continually relate my comments more broadly to other students' work in a more general sense.

A final word of caution is to gently, carefully protect the vulnerability of the student who is sharing her or his work. Using comments that underscore the future, such as, "As you move your project forward, you'll need to consider . . ." recognizes that it is a work in progress. This tone does not demean or send the message that "you forgot something . . . you didn't remember to . . . you forgot to consider that . . ."

CONCLUSION

To co-construct the classroom, we must be comfortable with our pliability and impressionability. There is a core of freedom that must be recognized before co-construction can happen, perhaps even a ragamuffin and barefoot state of mind for both the students and the faculty.

This embrace of co-construction is echoed by Azar Nafisi (2003) in her description of when she met with seven committed female students in the Islamic Republic of Iran to teach and learn together in her living room. Using forbidden Western classics, she described co-construction: I "selected a number of books to read, but I was prepared to let the class shape me; I was prepared for the violin to fill the void, and alter it by its music" (p. 28). For me, this comfort with co-construction has been a career-long journey to emerge, to become part of my history—but I am beginning to feel the shaping, enjoy the play, and hear the notes of the violin and the bells of freedom. And that is my wish for you.

QUESTIONS TO PONDER

1. To what extent do you agree with Bronowski's assertion that students must "bring a certain ragamuffin, barefoot irreverence to their studies?" Describe rationale for your perspective. What approaches do you/can you use to teach and learn with students who tend toward boldness and cheeky-ness?
2. Propose several ways that accountable talk can be encouraged in your teaching situation.
3. In what ways are students' names important to you? How might students' names be used advantageously? Disadvantageously? What connections can be made between using students' names in the educational setting to using names of colleagues in the practice setting?
4. Providing students with sample sentences, paragraphs, and papers is described in this chapter and elsewhere in this book. What assumptions underlie that technique? What other viewpoints may be possible?

REFERENCES

Giuliani, R. W. (2002). *Leadership.* New York: Hyperion.

Hoffman, E. (1989). *Lost in translation: A life in a new language.* New York: Penguin Books.

Lepp, M., & Zorn, C. R. (2002). Life circle: Creating safe space for education empowerment. *Journal of Nursing Education, 41*(9), 383–385.

Nafisi, A. (2003). *Reading Lolita in Tehran: A memoir in books.* New York: Random House.

CHAPTER 11

Creative Projects: "Could You Please Tell Us What You're Looking For?"

Carl Hammerschlag was asked by a Native American patient if he could dance. He shuffled his feet a bit and the patient said, "That's good." Realizing that there was some purpose to the patient's request, Carl asked him if he would dance as well. The patient adjusted his oxygen cannula and danced vigorously right there on his bed. Carl paused for a moment, then asked the patient if he could teach him to dance like that. The healer said, "I can teach you my steps, but you must hear your own music."

—Carl Hammerschlag

Through my years of teaching, I have usually assigned a creative project in my undergraduate and graduate courses. I use the term *creative project* loosely, referring to any student learning activity where creativity is explicitly required. Typically, I expect students to generate some product linked to course content that could be shared with others. The idea is that students will not write another straightforward, literature-based, scholarly paper to meet this requirement because they have ample experience with that already. At a less intense level, I request creativity as one of several requirements in a conventional learning activity; for example, I might ask students to be creative in their small group class presentations. Despite my repeated good intentions, however, I'm not convinced that the creative projects I assigned were as momentous, as learning-rich as I expected or hoped.

Admittedly, a few students kindly told me how much they benefited from my classes, but they rarely cited the creative project as an important part. And yes, with the creative project an occasional talented brilliance surfaced—a gifted student–artist weaving a wall hanging or a promising poet writing a profound piece. I reverently remember the stunning line drawing of a leaf that seemed to draw itself as the student hardly looked at her pencil and modestly murmured, "I just concentrate on *seeing* it." We all celebrated this, of course.

121

Mistakenly, however, my intent in incorporating creative projects in my early teaching was for the product to be art gallery worthy. Furthermore, because I didn't examine the teaching and learning aspects of creative activities, the results, from an education perspective, may have been mediocre at best. For many students, I suspect the learning resulting from project was sketchy and superficial, and the creative activity itself a humdrum drill, or perhaps an agonizing chore. Although the idea felt impressive, I was all thumbs and fraught with self-doubt. But since, I've learned a great deal from and about using creative projects because students repeatedly have asked, "Could you please tell us what you're looking for?"

The goal of this chapter is to help new faculty incorporate creative projects in their teaching. Three primary aspects are discussed: (1) personal experiences and musings, (2) conceptual characteristics of creativity, and (3) application to classroom teaching. Admirably, most novice teachers are motivated to "be creative," seeing this as one of the pleasurable aspects of teaching. For many, however, the prospect is daunting, their skills are minimal, and they receive little support from their colleagues. In fact, new faculty are often icily reminded that "creativity is frosting on the cake."

A NEWBIE'S ANEMIC ATTEMPTS

In the past, whenever I required a creative project and students would ask, "Could you please tell us what you're looking for?" I responded with a few measly words or evaded the question altogether. And I suspect the students spent hours anguishing over the answer on their own—perhaps *that* was the creativity, the innovation, unraveling yet another ambiguous impasse?

Most of the students didn't know how to begin, and I wasn't going to tell them. After all, wouldn't telling them dilute the creativity? Quite honestly, I didn't know how the students should begin either. Making matters worse, the students didn't know what I was looking for, and more than likely neither did I. Even if I did know, should I tell them? Does the teacher look for something in a creative project? In any case, doesn't discussing the requirements or evaluative criteria limit the creativity?

What's more, I disregarded, perhaps silently snubbed, the students' pleas of "I'm not creative. I can't draw or paint!" I found myself thinking: Why don't they just get on with it? What can possibly be so hard about doing a creative project? My impatience rankled, my edginess escalated, and as the creative project due date loomed, this "tell me—no, I can't tell you" cat-and-mouse game spiraled between the students and me.

Whether creativity was the stand-alone focus with a tangible outcome (i.e., the art gallery approach) or a component of a more traditional assignment, student worry and my ineptness at explaining the importance and meaning of the creative project were commonplace and shaded the whole venture. It has taken me a while, but I'm finally attending to the students' question "Could you please tell us what you're looking for?"

WHAT I'VE DISCOVERED

To begin, I must clarify my assumptions and describe what I've learned about creativity. Students, like all people, are creative; this ingenuity is one of our most remarkable resources and it must be cultivated in higher education. There is an innate human ability to be innovative, and students can create where there is a welcoming and sustaining learning environment. Margaret Wheatley (2001), an organizational scholar whose managerial study is grounded in biological systems, responded to the accusations that people are not creative and resistant to change with, "Could this possibly be true? Are we the only species—out of fifty million—that digs in its heels and resists? Or perhaps all those other creatures simply went to better training programs?" (p. 12).

Growing numbers of people call for creativity in our college graduates. Baccalaureate degree goals name creativity as an outcome. Business leaders demand creativity in their employees—not only in solving problems but in framing problems and they even go so far as to launch an "imagination award." Perhaps in health care we have not gone far enough; perhaps we have focused on solving problems and have not emphasized the need to creatively frame them, that is, to name, identify, describe, and examine their historical evolution. But that's another essay.

When students are interested in an issue or study issues that they see as critical in their personal or professional lives, their creativity immediately surfaces. The challenge for us as educators, then, is to determine what is meaningful for them.

To do that, I've discovered that we need to pay attention to what students talk about, what gives them energy, what makes them squirm or sit up. We need to teach and learn alongside them, and learn who they are, what charms them, what draws them. We must sit at the students' tables in the learning resource center, engage in their small group work meetings, and spend time at the back of our classrooms.

We must learn to pay attention to another's thoughts and methods as did the artist Vermeer when he met the teenaged housemaid, Griet, who became the image in *Girl with a Pearl Earring* in 1660s Holland (Chevalier, 1999, p. 5). When Vermeer first saw Griet in the scullery, she was arranging the vegetables as slices in a circular pie before tossing them into the soup pot. "Are they laid out in the order in which they will go into the soup?" Vermeer asked as he studied the circle sitting on the slab of wooden table.

"No, sir." But Griet could not say why she arranged the vegetables in this way. She simply set the vegetables as she felt they should be, but was too frightened to say so to a gentleman.

"I see you have separated the whites," Vermeer observed, indicating the turnips and onions. "And then the orange and the purple, they do not sit together. Why is that?" He picked up a shred of dark cabbage and a piece of carrot and shook them like dice in his hand.

After looking at her mother, who nodded slightly, Griet replied, "The colors fight when they are side by side, sir."

As educators, we won't learn *why* students arrange the vegetables as they do, or *how* they create the links that they pattern, or *what* they deem magic in their lives if we never enter the scullery—that is to say, if we stay in the margins or take the word of other faculty. In fact, it is tempting to be persuaded by others as they hastily label students in ways that brand them in negative and sweeping ways.

Several years ago, a faculty colleague of mine was exasperated with a student who was planning to take a semester's leave from the nursing program to work in health care in a developing country. The student, in her enthusiasm and unfamiliarity with such an endeavor, had not yet secured the necessary vaccinations and documentation required to travel in that geographic area and was scurrying for the faculty's help just days before her departure. This last-minute dashing about necessitated many thorny and convoluted phone calls, as well as pleading, on-the-spot meetings. In her annoyance, my colleague marked the student as "needy," a tag that stuck with the young woman for several semesters and among numbers of faculty. Thinking back, however, at age 20, I probably would not have preplanned all the travel requirements either and would also have frenzied hysterically at the last minute.

As it turned out, this student was extremely talented in many academic, humanitarian, and aesthetic ways, and she received multiple honors and awards by the time she completed the program. I dream for all students to be so "needy." (As I continue to mull this over, might it be that we, as the faculty, are really those who are needy?)

We know that labels for individual students often expand into labels for the entire class—the "contrary bunch," "the lot of them clinging to their cell phones." Always we must remain skeptical and hear those labels guardedly because it is those names that painfully pin students into categories. Instead, we need to hear what lures students, what fascinates them. We learn more when we are curious than we do when we are convinced. We learn how creativity can be stirred and integrated into higher education when we see and hear what *is* meaningful to students rather than predetermining what *should* be meaningful to them.

I've also discovered the power of creativity. When we express something, it is in a form that we understand; this expression translates the language of our soul. When we discover something, we see our spontaneous and free ideas and feelings in a painting, a poem, or a sculpture, often for the first time. Bibi Chen, the museum art collector in Amy Tan's *Saving Fish from Drowning* (2005), explains her first discovery of art: "My heart cavorted within shapes and shadows and splashes, in patterns, repetitions, and abruptly ending lines. My soul shivered in tiny feathered strokes, one eyelash at a time" (p. 31). The power of creativity, then, is the breakthrough, the jagged surface, the frolicking dance of the heart regardless of the limits, or perhaps because of the restrictions.

CREATIVITY AS A CONCEPT

Not only have I discovered the vigor of creativity, but I have also grown to understand it as a concept. To help readers release creative inhibition to support writing the natural way, Gabriele Rico (2000) summarizes Harry Broudy's classification of creative development: (1) innocent, creative expression, occurring from age 2 to 7, has few preconceived ideas about what should, ought, or must be done; (2) conventional expression, from age 8 to 16, is preoccupied with correctness, becomes more anxious, and loses spontaneity and originality; and (3) a reintegration of the innocent expression resulting in a cultivated, mature expression of creative impulses. That is, moving beyond the second stage requires us not to try harder, but to recultivate the wonder and improvisation from our childhood, and then join it to our learning, values, skills, and eagerness to grow.

Creativity is not simply either/or—you are creative or you're not. Sometimes we hastily and simply associate our left brain with logic and rationality and our right brain with artsy-crafty creativity. This dissection reinforces the either/or split, emphasizing that we are one and not the other. Unfortunately, this belief supports a person's notion that "I can't draw or paint—I'm not creative."

In actuality, as Rico (2000) describes, the creativity occurs when we fluctuate between the mind's ability to form the big picture and then to clarify and sequence the details. Our "Design" ability suggests pattern, connectedness, a whole, a scope and purpose, however tentative. Design focuses on the both/and, with its ambiguities and flow. In comparison, our "Sign" ability suggests parts, sequences, and separate pieces of information that can be noted. Either/or and discriminating characteristics are part of Sign. Yet, Design and Sign work collaboratively and are both essential for the creative process—it is not *either* Design *or* Sign. In that linkage, Design synthesizes and connects; Sign records features and differentiates. Creativity, then, is the ongoing vacillation between the two, continually "Sign-ing" and "Redesign-ing."

Although both Design and Sign are indispensable in our creative process, Rico maintains that we must begin with Design—the melody, and not the notes that compose the melody. As in the Native American healer's gentle chide to Carl Hammerschlag, Design is the music, and Sign is the particular dance steps.

Rico claims that when we begin with the rules imposed from without (as most of us were taught), the result is generally dreary and lifeless. Instead, she urges us to begin from within, awakening and extending our Design mind. Rico calls Design our neglected "stepchild in education" (p. 5). That neglected stepchild is our play, our improvisation, and our fantasy. That neglected stepchild is playing the edges, nudging and enlarging the boundaries.

BEGINNING TO MAKE IT A PRACTICE

So, after contemplating creativity within my teaching and learning, what have I learned? Or, as the students pressed, "what am I looking for?" The following before and after discussion of a creative project in a graduate course on nursing leadership sifts this out. Please be assured, however, that the "after" still needs more thought, more work, more Designing, Signing, and Redesigning.

As part of a required nursing leadership course in a master's program, I asked the students to each do a creative project. It was 25% of the course grade and due during the final class meeting. The other course assignments (in-class essay exam, scholarly paper, and professional class presentation) were traditional learning activities and I described my expectations for them in considerable detail.

For example, I distributed a topic list and sample essay questions prior to administering the essay exam and I made sample scholarly papers from previous classes available online. For the creative project, however, I listed only the following guidelines in the syllabus: (1) a personal reflection about the meaning of leadership as you move into a graduate-prepared nurse role, (2) substantive and sufficiently detailed, (3) clearly connected with course experience and course content, and (4) shared with the rest of the class in an informal way (3–4 minutes) during the last class meeting.

As described earlier, students were confused, anxious, and not at all keen about the project. And, in truth, I fumbled halfheartedly in offering feeble help. The students' projects were varied; collages were common, as were 3- to 4-page scrapbooks. The students' pithy comments shared at the final class meeting included little evidence of leadership theory or their role as master's-prepared nurse leaders. When I evaluated the projects, if the students created something or responded to something creative that they selected (for example, a well-known painting or poem) and made some comments about it in class (which they all did), they received a full 25% A grade for the assignment.

I'm reminded here about Thomas Edison's work late in his life when he was trying to develop a filament in his light bulb that would not instantly burn out. After months of still unsuccessful around-the-clock attempts by teams of people, his supervisor said something like, "Mr. Edison, I am sorry to say that we have done a thousand experiments, and it has all been for nothing." Edison retorted, "Nonsense, we now know a thousand ways in which it doesn't work!"

I have also learned some things that do not work for me and have made some changes that bolster the project's effectiveness. At a basic level, when student activities or assignments are new to students (i.e., they have had little practice with them previously), they need more, rather than less, discussion and guidelines. And yet, initially I provided substantial details about the essay exam, scholarly paper, and class presentation (all of which are familiar to college students) and scanty instruction for the creative project.

Now, I spend much more time in class discussing the project up-front before the students' unease rises. However, I've learned not to do this on the first day of class when all course syllabi are introduced, lives jam, and calendars over-flow. Even if a solitary eager student asks about it on the first day, I gently delay the discussion. Two or three weeks into the semester seems to be a good time to discuss it, beginning with, "Some of you are probably thinking about the creative project," or "In the past, students have worried about the creative project. Let's spend a little time talking about that now."

To begin, I underscore the progression of creativity as we age—moving from the innocent, to the conventional, and finally to the cultivated phase. Repeatedly, students describe themselves in the second phase, focused on correctness and conforming to external approval, with little inventiveness and loads of worry. At this point, the students and I smile as we recognize the conceptual location of their question "What have other students done for the project?" as being in the conventional phase.

Next, I discuss the third phase of creative development to provide a critical guideline for proceeding with the creative project. Revisiting the spontaneity of childhood and linking that imagination to an understanding and valuing of the leadership content is eye-opening for students. In this "ah-ha" moment, students are clear that it is this connection—the tie between the playful creativity of childhood and the learning and discovery of leadership—that must be unmistakable. A student comment might reflect this insight, "Oh, now I get it. I don't just get to finger-paint like when I was 4 years old—but I *can* finger-paint if that expresses my deepening grasp of leadership. And I need to learn more about the colors, strokes, and depth of finger painting so that I can use it more seriously. And I certainly am not going to worry about what the rest of the class thinks about my finger painting."

In my earlier experiences with the creative project, students frequently would become mired in their innocent childhood expression with barely a connection to in-depth course content. In such projects, then, they are unambiguously invited to move beyond the creative expression of childhood, through the preoccupation with correctness, and into a mature creative expression in the third phase. I stress also that this mature creative expression needs to be evident in their product as well as in their shared comments. That is, the wonder and innovation, as well as their learning about leadership in their master's-prepared nurse role, must be clear to others.

Building on the phases of creative development, I also highlight the Design and Sign components of creativity with the students. This dissuades some of the "I'm not creative" thinking. The essential quality of both cognitive processes not only demands, but also liberates graduate-level work. I encourage the students to (1) begin with Design—a whole idea or pattern about themselves as master's-prepared nurse leaders, grounded in one or more leadership theories, (2) examine the separate parts, the categorization, the sequencing within the idea to employ their Sign abilities, and (3) continue the process, using both components in tandem.

To help launch Design thinking, I suggest a few questions and ask the class as a group to brainstorm others: What am I learning about leadership? How is my leadership different now from when I completed my baccalaureate degree? How does my leadership compare to a character in a novel or a movie? Which leadership theory(s) appeal to me and why? A word of caution here: Be deliberate about Design by always studying the big-picture connections and purpose because students may exhibit a tendency to curl and twist in the detailed parts of Sign, which in its shadow side can also become the critic or the censor that stymies the process.

Finally, emphasize individual students' fascination. Sometimes they stew about choosing a medium for their creative expression and fall back on "I'm not creative." In this struggle, I propose that they consider what they have enjoyed doing in the past or a part of themselves that they would like to develop further. Providing examples of previous students' media such as dance routines, poetry, painting, quilting, gardening, photography, music, or clothing design, is helpful. I expect students to create their own project rather than to select someone else's creative expression. I stress that both innovative creation and their learning about the course content are essential to include.

I offer other guidelines that are helpful to the students: Begin early to spend some time thinking and creating the project—don't wait until the night before. At the same time, don't create the project at the start of the term because you need to be substantially immersed in the leadership content or your result will be scanty. Additionally, integrating culture, family, and personal or professional history will enrich the experience.

I wonder if the "nudge" concept described by Thaler and Sunstein (2008) might be helpful here and in other situations where we guide, question, and coach students to take their thinking to a higher level. Although I've not considered this intensely, I offer the possibility. The authors propose that a person called a *choice architect* organizes the context in which people make decisions. Recognizing that small and insignificant details can seriously influence people's choices, this architect may use social influences such as information, peer pressure, and priming to "channel" certain behaviors. Thaler and Sunstein focus their discussion on health, wealth, and happiness decisions, but might the nudge concept also be applied to learning and discovery?

By broadly linking the *choice architect* to education, then, the teacher as the architect can influence choices by arranging or constructing the environment that supports students' higher-level thinking. In the context of this chapter, the teacher facilitates the reintegration of childhood expressions with the students' new learning, values, and skills.

For example, can priming be used by the choice architect–educator? Using the stimulus notion, "priming" has its origin in older water pumps that required a dose of water to function properly. Might stellar role models be used more frequently, intensely, and effectively to prime current students? Perhaps describing the high-quality projects that students have done in the past (peer pressure) can nudge the current students. Or perhaps highlighting the (reasonably large) numbers of hours that previous students have used to prepare their project also nudges the current students. Might removing an obstacle such as an overwhelming paper length requirement or a massive minimum number of references required be used as a primer to channel a desired outcome, such as a more in-depth project? I will continue to mull over the nudge and invite you to do the same.

As the creative project has evolved, two additional considerations have been particularly helpful for me. First, I ask the students to submit a one-page written summary of the experience during their presentations on the last class day. This writing takes their thinking to a deeper level and encourages them to connect their innovation with the leadership content. As always, writing facilitates discovery. It also helps me remember each of the projects after class.

In addition, I plan ample time (30–45 minutes) for class discussion about the project (i.e., creativity development, Design/Sign abilities, personal meaning) sometime during the semester. Otherwise, if I provide only little bits of explanation as students are packing their bags at the end of class, they feel rushed and the hidden message is that the project is not important—it's merely more busywork. On the other hand, if I do all I can to emphasize the worth and magnitude of the activity, the students "hear" its centrality and meaning.

A preceptor colleague often requests students to submit a one-page proposal well ahead of the due date for a substantial or complex assignment. For example, 4 to 6 weeks before a 15-page paper is due, she requires a one-page outline that includes the major headings and subheadings, as well as three to five references. The one-pager is required (perhaps to pass the course) but is not graded with points or a letter grade. In this way, the students get started early and receive feedback on their topic selection and overall focus. The faculty, in turn, can present specific additional guidelines to help all students develop their work further after she has seen patterns of difficulty or areas that are thin or missing. This strategy could also be beneficial with the creative project. As usual, I've learned that providing students with specific and direct expectations even for a one-page proposal is essential.

CONCLUSION

The creative project is an opportunity for the students and for me to strike out on a voyage rather than to go out on tiny little trips. This voyage is part of rocking with the world as the actor-poet-musician-painter Viggo Mortensen describes: "To be an artist, you don't have to compose music or paint or be in the movies or write books. It's just a way of living. It has to do with paying attention, remembering, filtering what you see and answering back, participating in life" (10 questions, 2008, p. 9).

I am honored to recognize and encourage my own and others' paying attention and participating in life, to help us all move beyond flapping in the middle of the flock. In this vein, what I am looking for is for all students not to be limited in their goodness, but to begin to launch their greatness—just as a way of living.

QUESTIONS TO PONDER

1. Considering Broudy's classification of creative development into innocent, conventional, and reintegration, what commonalities do you as an

educator have with each of the 3 phases? What specific examples illustrate these commonalities?

2. What experiences have you had with creative activity as a student? Describe the experience from your student perspective. How would you characterize the teacher experience and perspective in that activity?

3. How might the Design and Sign approach be used in other areas of teaching, such as clinical education or evaluation of students?

4. When integrating creative activity into nursing education, what significant consequences are possible? In your current setting, are those consequences highly probable or less likely to occur?

REFERENCES

Chevalier, T. (1999). *Girl with a pearl earring.* New York: Penguin Putnam.

Rico, G. (2000). *Writing the natural way: Using right-brain techniques to release your expressive powers.* New York: Penguin Putnam.

Tan, A. (2005). *Saving fish from drowning.* New York: Ballantine Books.

10 questions. (2008). *Time, 172*(26), 9.

Thaler, R. H., & Sunstein, C. R. (2008). *Nudge: Improving decisions about health, wealth, and happiness.* New Haven, CT: Yale University Press.

Wheatley, M. (2001, Spring). We are all innovators. *Leader to Leader, 20,* 11–21.

Nursing Education as Liberal Education

CHAPTER 12

Teaching Life, Not Teaching Work

Cautious, careful people always casting about to preserve their reputation and social standing, never can bring about a reform.

—Susan B. Anthony

"And the final product of our training must be neither a psychologist nor a brickmason, but a man" (DuBois, 1986, p. 423). This W. E. B. DuBois quote is as germane for us today as it was in 1903 when written by one of the century's greatest African American educator–scholars. Over a hundred years later, our aim in nursing education still begs the question: Are we preparing a nurse or preparing a person? By adapting a related DuBois assertion, we must also ask ourselves: To what extent do we simply "teach work," or beyond that, how does our nursing education "teach life"?

The goal of this book is to help us move beyond teaching the work of nursing and draw us closer to teaching life with nurses. I trust that the book's major units—knowing the self as teacher, examining relationships with students, and describing teaching practices—will uphold new and emerging faculty as they realign closer to that goal.

Shifting the preparation of nurses away from a rigid professional studies focus that emphasizes workforce development carries us past teaching work and nearer to teaching life. Repositioning nursing education as liberal education inspires this shift and invites essential and exhaustive discourse. I propose the following to launch this dialogue: (1) moving beyond compliance in health care, (2) discussing the shadow side of present-day nursing education, and (3) understanding three dimensions of nursing education as liberal education.

BEYOND COMPLIANCE IN HEALTH CARE

In her recent book *Bait and Switch: The (Futile) Pursuit of the American Dream*, journalist Barbara Ehrenreich (2005) went undercover. This was a covert experience similar to the one in her previous look at minimum-wage jobs in *Nickel and Dimed* (2001). This time, however, she became an unemployed job-seeking professional, a role she assumed to study terminated (or soon-to-be terminated) white-collar workers' lives.

One of the many lessons Ehrenreich learned in her concealed position in *Bait and Switch* was the vast pervasiveness of an "inward-looking" culture in corporate America. In this culture, the boss is the most important customer and the emphasis is on employee likeability, being a team player, and a personality "that is relentlessly cheerful, enthusiastic, and obedient . . . requisite personality traits even trump intelligence" (p. 228). She found this corporate culture insisted on employee upbeatness and compliance and she described these as qualities of subordinates, of servants rather than masters, of women (traditionally, anyway) rather than men.

While she sought a professional position, advice on "dumbing down" her résumé surfaced everywhere. As a result of these short-sighted, limiting corporate characteristics, Ehrenreich maintains that a generalized culture of incompetence is the stunning and devastating consequence.

To the degree that our healthcare culture is similarly inward looking, demands compliance, and likewise is "addicted to untested habits, paralyzed by conformity, and shot through with magical thinking" (Ehrenreich, 2005, p. 226), healthcare quality decays. In that culture of incompetence, a patriarchal system drives nurses while they wispily submit to corporate standards rather than those of the profession. The nurse prepared for life, and not merely prepared for work, is able to open a reform in health care, which is currently permeated by a culture of incompetence.

Untested habits and paralytic conformity reveal themselves in all the crevices of our healthcare system. It was a Midwest-humid, stifling July afternoon. I was volunteering at a local pantry distributing food and other essentials to individuals and families who come weekly by city bus, bicycle, or car. After standing in the dripping swelter waiting for the pantry door to open that day, the people crowded into the small waiting room. A slow ceiling fan groaned to stir the stuffy air.

In the food pantry, the distribution process is deliberate and measured, spiked with a hint of power distinction. On a small pinch of paper, the people who call at the pantry write down items they select from a master list of food and essentials, as well as the number of people in their household. As each person's number is called, a volunteer uses that handwritten order form to fill a cardboard box with items from the large storage room shelves, and then returns the filled box to the person.

I completed an order that afternoon from a young mother with a crying infant in her arms and two tired, sweaty, and squabbly toddlers at her side. I worried about the "one adult, five children" in the upper left-hand corner of her list. Four rolls of toilet paper, three dozen diapers, and six jars of baby food were written on her request, none of which were on the near-sacred master list posted on the waiting room wall.

The scribbled items on her list pleaded soundlessly, "I know these aren't on the master and this is not allowed, but I really need them, so if you could just slip them in the box, please?" My heart hurdled as I saw the young woman and her petition for the nonsanctioned items.

Trying to be invisible, I slid all the items she requested in her box. At that moment, another volunteer noticed the additional things, muscled over to me, and screeched, "We're not supposed to give extra things away. If we do this for one person, we have to do it for everybody. The supervisor told us this before he left. Didn't you hear? You have to put the toilet paper and diapers back on the shelf!"

Standing in the storage room doorway, the young mother heard everything as she rocked her sniffling baby. Long bedraggled bangs veiled her downcast eyes and disgrace melted her face. I muttered and foamed, my blood in bubbles, "I don't have the heart to say no to this woman." Yet, with throat clogged and strangling hands, I yanked the baby food and the paper products out of the box and spinelessly returned them to the storage room shelf.

Of course, I acknowledge the noble food pantry mission and its virtuous, long-standing contribution to the community. And yes, on that steamy July afternoon as I put the items back on the shelf, I was compliant, marinating in holiness, perhaps. Nonetheless, I must attend to the malevolence and hypocrisy I still feel from denying those items. Why was I so pathetic and feeble, so puny and scrawny? Why did I conform to "do the work"?

Julie Otsuka (2002) portrays a similar, but much more painful and enraging incident in her novel *When the Emperor Was Divine*. She described a Japanese American woman reclassified as an enemy alien in 1942, uprooted, and sent to a grimy internment camp in the Utah desert. She packed her household, item by item, "and the woman, who did not always follow the rules, followed the rules" (p. 9).

At one time or another, most of us have been the young mother, the screeching colleague, the dithering volunteer, the decent yet shallow supervisor enforcing or making the rules, or perhaps even someone exiled following the rules. Comparable episodes repeat themselves a thousand-fold in our broken healthcare system. Because of these incidents and the millions of casualties they strew about, nurses must be prepared for more than the work of nursing or there is no hope for change.

In their preparation, nurses' intelligence cannot be trumped by cheerfulness and obedience. Neither can a scientific, evidence-based practice be trumped by paralytic conformity nor can a compassionate humanity be trumped by hollow policy and procedure. Nursing education as liberal education holds promise for that decisive preparation, and many of our programs and faculty are striking out on that path. The acumen and principled conviction of Susan B. Anthony beckon us: Cautious, careful people always casting about to preserve their reputation and social standing never can bring about a reform.

Yet, despite our audacity, there still may be a shadow side to our education systems and what we do within those systems. These shadows implore our analysis.

SHADOW SIDE OF NURSING EDUCATION

Often a liberal nursing education is seen as a "building on" approach—where general education (GE) is one brick, and nursing coursework is another brick in the wall of higher education. This is often translated as a distinct division: Over there, on that side of campus or at that university is "liberal," and over here, on this side of campus or in our college is "nursing" or "professional."

In their brave discussion in *Declining by Degrees: Higher Education at Risk*, Hersh and Merrow (2005) propose that the professional fields see the *value* in liberal education but, unfortunately, do not see it as their *responsibility*. For example, we declare that someone else on the other side of campus or over in Arts and Sciences or in the Humanities Building teaches the liberal education and I teach nursing. Or, at the end of a worn-out day, we protest in despondence, "I have all I can do to teach nursing—the rest is not my job."

Hersh and Merrow (2005) probe further, "If disciplines and departments are not considered responsible for the broad outcomes of liberal education, who is?" (p. 68). They charge that "the academy has lowered its sights for liberal education from the entire college curriculum to that small fraction of the undergraduate experience known as general education" (p. 69).

Might it be, then, that the liberal education structure of our nursing program is receding, shrinking away, exposing the pebbles and rubble of disconnect? Modifying Hitchens's (2001) suggestion to a young contrarian, we must ask ourselves, "What do they [the students] or we know of nursing, who *only nursing* know?" (p. 105). Without nursing as a liberal education, we know only a shaving or a splinter.

Often we even illustrate this disconnect between nursing and liberal education or GE in our nursing curricular models and organizing frameworks. We sketch building blocks, pyramids, stairways, and ladders to illustrate nursing education; one step in the stairway is natural sciences, one step is humanities, one step is nursing, and one step may be service learning.

It is assumed, then, that when the student climbs to the top of the stairway or clambers all the ladder rungs, a liberally educated nurse graduates. Maybe this assumption is another example of what Em Bevis (Bevis & Watson, 2000) depicts as the null curriculum: the curriculum that does not exist, although we say it does (often in colorful language and with exquisite and creative graphics). That is, we declare that nursing courses built on or added to GE courses or other curricular requirements result in a liberally educated nurse; however, that may not always be the situation.

In the minds and practices of many students and faculty, nursing or professional study is distinctly separated from GE and liberal education. Beyond this view of separateness, and even more troublesome, there is an implicit notion that GE is flimsy, even worthless. I have often heard faculty and students refer to "getting their GE courses out of the way," breathing an audible sigh of relief when that has been accomplished. Presumably, then students can get to the real reason they came to college. To me, this outlook denotes GE as fluff, another hoop to jump through, and not critical to nursing education.

I must own up. I also have made these same comments, but I am trying to be more meticulous in reframing nursing as liberal education in my discussions with colleagues and in the way I teach and learn with students.

In addition to this building on model where nursing courses are added to GE courses, there also are other ways that building occurs in nursing education. In some systems, there is an increasing rate of transfer courses, where students hop from campus to campus citing location, tuition costs, GPA advantages, and changes in major as their rationale. Certainly, these are understandable reasons to change colleges, but this approach may add to the "brick-by-brick" affair.

Furthermore, in some areas high school students are taking more advanced placement (AP) courses. Again, financial considerations are completely reasonable and will become more substantial as public funding for higher education erodes.

Yet, to what extent is there a liberal education focus for the teenager in these classes? For example, how are 16- or 17-year-olds in AP English helped to connect their writing skills to other college-level coursework—appreciating literature, analyzing the culture of a healthcare organization, untangling issues of privilege, and learning about themselves?

In my view, the liberally educated individual must be able to critically analyze. I'm reminded of Trimble's (1975) description of writing a *critical analysis* compared with a *plot summary*. In this classic little helpful writing handbook, Trimble presents a plot summary example as a collection of highlights of the Vietnam War that contain no thesis, no point of view, written in the past tense. In a plot summary, the goal is to describe; think "what." In contrast, Trimble explains a critical analysis of the Vietnam War would contain answers to the following questions: How did the United States enter the war, why did they stay, and what effects did this have on the people? In a critical analysis writers take a point of view, support a daring thesis, make sense of something, explain and evaluate, and stick their necks out. In analysis, writers interpret, think "how" and "why," and help the reader discover.

Are high school AP English students capable of writing and thinking as critical analysts? Have the students made the concurrent discoveries to support this depth of analysis, or is the AP course designed to earn college credit but remain an isolated class with little foundation or bracing from other learning? For the high school students in AP courses and the transfer students, who is teaching critical analysis? Who is integrating learning? Who is teaching life?

In all of these building approaches to higher education, students are cobbling together their college education in ways that may not result in a liberally educated nurse prepared for life. This cobbling morphs into an assembly line where students, as robots, pick the nut or bolt that their degree demands off the moving belt. The cobbling can be a cafeteria approach where students push their lunch tray along and select a course or a learning experience a la carte, as they count calories and credits and add grams and grades. In these assembly lines and cafeteria lines, there may be a sequence among the selected items, a building on, but the connections are loose or even imperceptible. More often, the items are detached from each other, with little or no interface among them.

In place of such building programs, I propose that students savor a fine dining experience where all the flavors of classes and learning experiences are integrated, blended with tight connections, changed by each other. That is, the wine augments the entree and coffee enhances dessert, making for a transformative evening.

Randy Pausch, professor of computer science at Carnegie Mellon University in Pittsburgh, Pennsylvania, wrote *The Last Lecture* (Pausch & Zaslow, 2008) before he died of pancreatic cancer. Someone once asked him, "What can schools do to help students dream bigger?" He replied, "All universities ought to do a better job of encouraging students to take courses outside of their major. Dreams come from broadening your horizons and rubbing elbows with different kinds of people." The crux is in the "rubbing elbows"; that is, where and when the connections are made, the transformative evening occurs.

Perhaps the building on approach has been our conventional wisdom, our conventional education, but where and how is integration accomplished? How do we help students rub elbows? Education for nurses must be blended, merged, mingled, and integrated. It is not a brick-by-brick affair, where a high school teacher or each professor on a college or university campus or each type of nursing education program lays a unique brick. Too often the result is little more than a collection of bricks on the graduate's transcript: bricks as courses, programs, or degrees.

These add-on approaches may be some of the dark shadows, the shade in the bigger picture of our nursing education system. There also may be shadows closer to home, more locally, within our programs, among our faculty, and even skulking inside our classrooms.

David Whyte (1994) describes education and how it influences the soul of corporate America. His statement both sickens and outrages me: "Our education has been bent toward . . . drying us out, tidying us up, and making us presentable for the great economic system that awaits us" (pp. 289–290). At a level nearer to the student and teacher and equally as heartrending, he argues that students are told that much of who they are, their self-identity, is not allowed in the classroom, particularly "the parts that think for themselves" (p. 290). Then, as employees later in life, Whyte insists, "These same parts of us stay out in the parking lot while we climb out of the car in the morning and head toward the revolving door of the building. The person left out in the car is often a part we once treasured: a person awestruck with wonder, ripe with the dumbest question, and thirsting to learn" (p. 290).

Horrifying as is Whyte's description, it demands that we ask the tough questions and struggle with our responses. To what extent do we insist that nursing students leave part of who they are at the classroom door in our effort to dry them out and tidy them up? How do we receive all the students, warts and all? What do we do with the nursing students who think for themselves? In what ways do we reward niceness and compliance while we penalize "dumb questions"? How do we label students as "needy" (how I do loathe that label)? How do we rejoice when a class needs only a whisper of our attention, as if teaching was not linked with attention, and the less attention we have to give, the better for us?

As these questions have been raised in dozens of faculty meetings I've attended, there frequently is a "isn't this terrible? No, not me, never . . ." sort of response. Or the dialogue is reframed as the fault of the students: "*They* just don't study enough. *They're* employed too many hours. The *students* now sure are different from when I was in school." Or we begin to design meaningless (or perhaps even draconian or destructive) rules to "dry them out and tidy them up" such as dress codes for class and skills labs that are over the edge, or brutal penalties for late assignments, while we take 4 to 6 weeks to return their graded work. Why is it so difficult to turn the mirror on ourselves, to consider how we teach and learn with students?

And then we must look down the road at that inward-looking healthcare corporation. Remembering that sweltering July afternoon in the food pantry, I am called to face the part of me I left in the car, the one that would have challenged the compliance that propelled my response. How commonly do nurses leave their wonder, their questions of suspicion and skepticism, their thirst to learn in the car in the parking lots as they head toward the revolving doors of our healthcare system?

Unquestionably, convenience, simplicity, economy, and comfort have cast some of the shadows in nursing education. Maybe getting admitted to a college or university, earning a degree, and securing a high-paying job have become too much the center stage for some legislators, parents, and students. Although momentous strides have shaped our nursing education history, too frequently our graduates are not liberally educated and, instead, are becoming advantaged citizens who do not understand a disadvantaged place. They may be prepared as nurses for the work of nursing, but they are not liberally educated as people for life. Quality health care for all and global citizenship demand the latter.

Let's pause and revisit DuBois's assertions. Against the backdrop of an inward-looking healthcare system that prizes compliance and yet lacks health, care, and system, as well as some lurking shadows in our nursing education programs, we ask: Are we preparing a nurse or a person? And further, are we teaching work or teaching life? I reaffirm nursing education as liberal education so that we can help prepare a person and teach life.

NURSING EDUCATION AS LIBERAL EDUCATION

So, what is nursing education as liberal education? I would like to conclude this unit and this book with some ideas. In truth, I hope that this conclusion is not an ending but a beginning. Although I cannot detail the direction of this continuing conversation, I am convinced that it must carry on and believe that new and emerging nursing faculty will seize the lead. To open the discussion, I propose that nursing education as liberal education is art, agency, and growth, and I have invited Drs. Lee Shulman, Maxine Greene, and John Dewey to join us. Let's begin the dialogue.

Nursing Education as Liberal Education Is Art

Dr. Shulman, you've devoted your life to teaching, learning, and learning to teach. As a basic premise, you've maintained that "to the extent that teaching is an art, its practice requires at least three forms of knowledge: knowledge of rules, knowledge of particular cases, and knowledge of ways to apply rules to cases" (Shulman, 2004, p. 175).

Of course, one could easily tie this idea to nurse educators, but if I may, Dr. Shulman, I'd like to link your view to nurses themselves. In that link, I suggest that a liberally educated nurse is a nurse–artist—one who knows the rules, knows the cases, and knows the most appropriate (best way) to apply the rules. Through a limited professional studies workforce development preparation, nurses know the rules. Historically, these rules emanated from tradition and authority figures; more recently, nursing research also confirms some of these rules and principles.

But simple knowledge of the rules does not make a nurse–artist. Knowing the rules may help the nurse handle what is familiar, address problems that are given, manage what is established. More distressingly, simply knowing the rules may paralyze us into conformity and freeze us in untested habits. At the food pantry, I knew the rules—actually, I needed a snarly reminder—but those rules petrified me into compliance. So, nursing education that concentrates on rules is not a liberal education. Is my extrapolation reasonable and fair-minded thus far, Dr. Shulman?

Beyond knowing the rules, a liberally educated nurse knows the particular cases and knows how to apply the rules to them. A liberal education—an integration of many disciplines—is essential to an introductory understanding of the human condition (i.e., the cases) across time and cultures. This is the key. The human condition begs us to unravel what it means to be human, people's attitudes toward life, how humans respond and what they value, how humans learn, and how they interact with each other.

To the extent that we curtail or lose that unraveling, our nursing education teeters on the verge of becoming trade schooling. For example, in learning about epidemics a liberally educated nursing student must study the microbiology of the culprit organism, the current available prevention methods, and the technique of their administration. However, a liberally educated nursing student also must have a broader understanding of the human condition that converges around epidemics. This human condition includes the history of epidemics, the responses of individuals and societies to them, as well as the complexity of lifestyles, environment, education, economy, food sources, politics, gender roles, wars and violence, and world religions. This convergence becomes the "particular case" of an epidemic.

Only after understanding particular cases, as it were, can nurses apply rules or research-generated principles with individuals, families, or communities as clients. Yes, the rules and principles ground the decisions that are made in providing nursing care, but a liberal education helps us learn what meaning rules and principles have for clients and how they can or must be modified, usually without doing away with the rules completely. Only then is nursing an art.

Dr. Shulman, I'd like to make one final twist on your idea, if I may. Knowing how to apply the rules as part of a liberal education requires also that we know the self.

A liberal education helps unify the person, the nurse who is experiencing, with the subject of that experience, the client situation. This unity between the nurse and the client situation must be revered and treated as whole. It is part of knowing the self. Exploring this unity is momentous, and as liberal education teachers, we honorably penetrate that discovery as co-learners with the students.

Too often, we merely intellectualize the experience students have with clients; that is, we urge students to examine clinical data and consult research articles to answer questions. Intellectualizing the experience keeps it "out there." Examining data and consulting research are necessary, of course, but we cannot stop there.

We also must help students learn about themselves—their feelings and growth, the context in which they find themselves, and the connections they are making as a result of the nursing care they provide. The experience students are having is part of them; the experience must enter the students. As faculty in liberal nursing education, we need to help students mine the human encounter. We merge previous courses, academic and community experiences, as well as the different spheres of students' own lives to help them explore the unity between themselves and the client situation. It is in this learning about the self that the nurse learns more about the rules, particular cases, and how to apply the rules. It is in this learning that the nurse becomes the nurse–artist.

To illustrate the unity between the self and the client situation, and also what it means for the liberal nurse educator, Dr. Shulman, I'd like to tell you about a personal experience. I was a 20-year-old nursing student learning about grieving and coping with death and dying.

It was the early 1970s and Kübler-Ross's grief stages were the hot topic. I learned the stages, as we all did at that time, and "applied" them to an elderly man with liver cancer and his wife whom I cared for in my clinical experience. They were the focus of the required 40-page nursing care plan paper. I suspect my intellectualizing about grief was somewhere in the A/B range because I learned a little about the client and his wife and their grieving (the rules, this particular case, and some application), but the experience was "out there."

Regrettably, in that course I didn't study how I related to that experience. Consequently, I learned little about myself.

However, it was in another course that same semester where, in fact, that single clinical experience became part of me and I learned much more about myself. In this course, a teacher wholly focused on liberal education prompted me to uncover how I related to caring for that dying man.

This teacher helped me write an "on my mind" essay in which the writer takes an idea that's been on his or her mind and delves into it and digs around. This single idea can be what you discuss or would like to discuss with your roommate, what you think about when you're walking to campus or driving the car, or what you wish would simply go away. This type of essay, the professor taught us, is "going deeper and deeper, rather than skimming the surface of many ideas. In this essay, you want to get to the roots of one idea, and uncover each root tenderly, relishing what it teaches you."

Today I realize that this professor was helping me learn about "rootedness." Dr. Shulman, you also described rootedness and attached it to learning. Liberal education, you said, "is mostly and most importantly *rooted* . . . the liberally educated person understands that there are roots, there are beginnings, there is a genesis, an evolution to ideas" (Shulman, 2004, p. 407).

So, what was on my mind while I cared for the dying man and his wife? What was the idea that just wouldn't go away?

One deep and dark December in their early years of marriage my parents lost a daughter named Celia 10 days after she was born. Because the gravedigger did not have special equipment to prepare a burial place in the frozen earth of northeastern Wisconsin, my sister's body was stored through the winter. She waited for spring in a tiny coffin in the basement of the mausoleum in the village cemetery back of beyond. Every Sunday after the church service, my parents would stop at the mausoleum. Barely 24 years old, my mother crept alone into that musty mournful basement to visit my sister in her small coffin while my dad minded their other two baby children in the car outside. It wasn't until mid-April when the days lengthened and the ground thawed that Celia could finally be buried.

I learned about that miserable winter from my mother years later, when I was probably 10 or 12 years old. After tearfully stumbling back to my bedroom, I spent months, perhaps years, sorrowfully imagining my young mother's grief all those blurry bleak Sunday mornings as she stood alone and caressed Celia's coffin, her tears dripping onto its cold metal cover. To this day, when I see Celia's miniature gravestone in our family plot, that dreadful and desolate image returns.

Today my mother is 91 years old, still walks to that same cemetery at least biweekly, and cleans up the faded artificial flowers strewn about most of the graves every spring. She actually saves all the flowers in her garage where they are jammed floor to ceiling, but that's another story about stewardship, poverty and the Depression, recycling, and global warming. Now, with a gritty spirit and a peaceful heart, my mother minces no words in her customary bluntness, "I know more people in the cemetery than I know living in the village." And one of those people in the cemetery is her own beloved baby Celia.

In writing that essay around my mother's experience, I opened some beginnings, tenderly uncovered the roots. To this day, I relish what that thinking and writing process taught me. I studied family relationships (my own and as described in theory), parents' grieving their loss of a child (again, my own and as described in the literature), causes of death in the early 1940s, burial practices, and legislation related to winter burials. Incidentally, state law now requires that winter burials be available in all cemeteries in Wisconsin so that grieving is not unnecessarily prolonged. In unearthing that genesis, I also discovered Russian poet Alexander Pushkin's lines: *But now I know, while beauty lives / So long will live my power to grieve.*

Needless to say, in the "on my mind" essay I recalled my mother's grief, but I actually examined my own grief and learned more about myself, my depths and my ghosts, my burdens and my gifts. Because of that liberal education experience, I united my encounter with the dying man and his wife with who I am.

As a result, Dr. Shulman, I learned a little about the rules around the grieving process and applying them to particular cases, I learned more about the human condition, and I learned a great deal about being a nurse–artist.

Guidelines for an "on my mind" essay are presented in Exhibit 12-1. Although, roughly speaking, the guidelines might be syllabus-ready, they are simply intended to provide the new nurse educator with a place to begin.

As can be seen in Exhibit 12-1, the writing process for the "on my mind" essay is divided into two phases. A multiple phase approach to any writing assignment helps students begin well before the final due date, prevent academic dishonesty, emphasize the paper's significance, and provide opportunity for faculty or peer feedback. Peer feedback can be extremely valuable; however, I've learned that peers benefit from being taught a specific focus. Providing the peers with 3–4 questions to address will help them be more beneficial to the writer. First, feedback can focus on idea development and clarity, organization, and thoroughness; second, the feedback might focus on grammar, word choice, sentence structure, and the like.

Nursing Education as Liberal Education Is Agency

It may seem more obvious to invite Dr. Maxine Greene (2001) to the previous dialogue about nursing education, liberal education, and art. As a philosopher and an aesthetics-in-education scholar, she has been renowned as knowing or having known just about everyone who was anyone in the world of art.

Begging your pardon, Dr. Greene, I'd prefer instead to draw on some of your ideas about agency in our dialogue here. What is exceptional about your look

Exhibit 12-1

Guidelines for an "On My Mind" Essay in Nursing Education
The purpose of this essay is to study an experience or an idea that has recently been "on your mind." For this study, select an experience you've had in clinical with a patient, family, or healthcare staff in the organization. Or you might choose an idea that has been percolating for some time, such as a technique that you think could be done differently, either in clinical or on campus, or a viewpoint that you've heard with which you disagree. This experience or idea is one that keeps coming back to you, one that you just can't seem to "shake off"—it might be one that is unsettling for you or that has affected you significantly in some way.

In writing the essay, you will develop skill in learning about something more deeply, going back to its roots, and connecting yourself with that idea. All of these skills are essential in helping you think like a leader.

Phase 1
Provide a 15-minute class time for the students to begin their essay. After introducing the purpose, prompts can be used to help students hand-write their beginning draft in class as a free-write. Encourage the students to write as much as possible responding to one of the following prompts, without taking their pens off their paper and without attention to grammar, word choice, or sentence structure: (1) "I've been thinking about something that happened with a patient the other day. I actually told some friends about it, but I don't think they really got it. What happened is that . . ." (2) "On the unit I see other nurses do this all the time. No one seems to question this yet I'm not sure if it really works or not. What I'm seeing is that . . ." or (3) "In my night class in (e.g., religion or women's studies), the professor said that . . . I'm not sure I totally agree and I know my parents certainly would not. Actually I don't think I understand fully what was said but it was something like . . ."

Phase 2
In a 5–6 page typed scholarly paper, please address the following 3 components. Be as specific as possible and provide examples to illustrate your points.
• How does the experience or idea you selected relate to your childhood, adolescence, or any previous life event or situation? In other words, how does something in your earlier life link with the idea you selected for this paper? Begin by considering why you selected the topic for the paper (approx. 2 pages).
• Relate your experience or idea to 2–3 discussions in the professional literature. In this section, compare the similarities and differences between your experience/idea and those of the referenced authors (approx. 2 pages).
• Describe your conclusions. How is your thinking changing ("I used to think that . . . but now I think that . . .)? In what areas are you still puzzled? If you were writing a second paper about this topic, what would it include? (approx. 2 pages)

at agency is that you've interwoven this concept with the ideas of feeling and passion. And in that interweaving, you've positioned agency as a core of liberal education. Now I see that is the aesthetician in you.

You've described agency as the "power to choose and to act on what is chosen . . . a willingness to take initiatives, to pose critical questions . . . to embark, whenever opportunities arise, on new beginnings" (Greene, 2001, p. 110). I'd like to add that inherent in this choosing and acting, though, is the belief that there is yet an unknown, a possibility. A belief that our story won't be foretold, instead it will unfold. That is, before we can believe we have the power to choose and to act, we must believe that someone else doesn't already have it all figured out—that the story hasn't already been foretold.

Dr. Greene, I'd like to describe an example to show you what I mean. In using the usual case study as a traditional teaching strategy we may already have predicted the correct answer to the questions. Typically, we create a clinical case to illustrate some significant points we're teaching, and then we pose several preidentified questions about that case for the students to answer. Often we present the case and then ask the students to answer the questions while they work with a partner or in small groups and while we take a break. We may even do this exact case study in the exact same way with the exact same questions semester after semester.

Truth be told, I've done my share of foretelling in this way. This pedagogy shuffles close to dullness if we expect the students simply to figure out what we already have jotted down on our tattered answer sheet. Figuring out the one right answer for each question obliterates the power to choose and to act on what is chosen—the story already has been foretold. Maybe this is another instance when students feel like seals in training?

An alternative may be to use the case study approach, but to pose only one question after the case is presented. Following that, we might ask for student response, and then create another observation, piece of information, or second question based on their response. Our expertise about the case helps us design these observations, bits of additional information, and questions. Those additions, along with the students' responses, all become part of the developing case. Continuing that type of cycle or similar unfolding subtly nudges the learners closer to believing that they have power to choose and to act. This alternative urges students to integrate many disciplines and probe the rootedness of the case. What's more, this is in closer harmony with nursing practice and is much more dynamic and fun.

Here's a quick and simple example of an unfolding case that could be used in the classroom to lift the students' sense of agency. In this case, a nurse is teaching Mr. Ahmden, a 70-year-old man who is being discharged with chronic congestive heart failure (CHF) after his fifth hospitalization in 8 months.

Your opening question might be, "What is the primary action that Mr. Ahmden can do to prevent recurrent hospital admissions for CHF in the future? Discuss the rationale for your response." Students' responses may include monitoring (e.g., observing weight gain, finger swelling with tightening jewelry rings, or ill-fitting shoes), dietary changes, or more accurate medication management. Hearing students' rationale will present the opportunity for affirmation and clarification.

After the students respond about the primary action, you then may offer further information about Mr. Ahmden's situation, such as lack of a bathroom scale, vision impairment, minimal English language skills, frequent dining out and alcohol use, current lab results, distinct food preferences, immigrant status from an East African country, lack of prescription drug coverage, and/or his life at home with his wife who has Alzheimer's disease. You might select specific information based on your knowledge of the students, what review is necessary, and the rationale they provided as their first response.

Posing a second question continues the case development: "Now, with the additional information you have and as the discharging RN, what single question is most important for you to ask Mr. Ahmden?" The case progresses as you provide the answer to the students' question (on Mr. Ahmden's behalf) and then pose another question or offer more information. In this way, students realize that the questions and answers are not all canned beforehand. The students and you become active agents in this patient's nursing care.

My apology for that bit of digression, Dr. Greene—I now return to the feelings that you acknowledged are part of agency. Agency is being skeptical, puzzling over assumptions and values, knowing that things aren't always what they seem, and asking questions.

A student once divulged how tricky, even terrifying it was for her to ask questions of an "authority" (e.g., teachers, her boss at the fast-food restaurant who was about 5 years younger than her, older students in her classes, and even her boyfriend). She described "not wanting to rock the boat. I just want to keep peace." It was as though this student tried to live molded to the smallest space possible. She could be portrayed as having no place to stand—she was all perch. Agency recoils from being a perch; agency claims a place to stand.

In contrast to this feeling of transparency that often hinders one's agency, other emotions are also intermingled with agency that actually carry it forward. Dr. Greene, you advise us that the uncertainty and inquiry that compel us to ask and puzzle in fact mandate a love of the question. That is, we must care for the skepticism and the doubt we feel, not turn our back on our confusion and distrust.

You cited the poet Rainer Maria Rilke's advice to a young student at the Military Academy of Vienna who was discouraged by the prospect of military life (published as *Letters to a Young Poet* in 1934). In one letter, Rilke reminded his correspondent how critical it was "to be patient toward all that is unsolved in your heart and to try to love the questions themselves like locked rooms and like books that are written in a very foreign tongue . . . live everything. Live the questions now" (Greene, 2001, p. 76).

From Rilke, therefore, we learn that loving and living the question cultivate the uncertainty and inquiry. In true elder/adviser style (admittedly, the "elder" Rilke was only 27 years old when the letters to the 19-year-old Franz Kappus began in 1902), he urges his reader to "try" to love the questions, wisely recognizing that honoring or loving the question is also a challenge that doesn't come simply.

Sandy Tolan in *The Lemon Tree* (2006, p. 253) echoes an even more crushing emotional struggle to speak, to voice, to pose the questions. At a most grim occasion in that historical narrative, Tolan cites Gideon Levy's October 17, 2004, column titled "Killing Children Is No Longer a Big Deal." In the column Levy, an Israeli columnist, reviews statistics from the Israeli-Palestinian conflicts, particularly the violence that has destroyed many Palestinian children. He writes, "With horrific statistics like this, the question of who is terrorist should have long since become very burdensome for every Israeli. Who would have believed that Israeli soldiers would kill hundreds of children and that the majority of Israelis would remain silent?"

I cannot envision a call to agency that could be more potent than Levy's entreaty. On a daily basis, as liberally educated nurses and nurse educators we must ask ourselves: "About what are we silent? Who will bewail us as they face our memory—can you believe they remained silent?"

Agency is about ending silence, claiming a place to stand; it is that agency that initiates the reconstruction of health care. Dr. Greene, you describe how agency is activated at an early age: "You can usher a child into a theater or museum, encourage, explain, tempt, support. But children must discover a sense of their own agency if the particular work of art is to come alive; they must make their own use of what has been taught" (Greene, 2001, p. 137).

It is obvious, then, that as nursing faculty we design or shape environments that awaken agency, but the discovery comes from within students. However, we have a distinct duty to help them make use of what has been taught.

This "making use" doesn't just happen. This making use needs more than a collection of bricks on students' transcripts. Making use is helping students integrate, mingle, and blend their learning experiences to learn more about themselves and the human condition. At the center of a nursing education as liberal education, in all that we do with students we must help them grasp the power to choose and to act on their choices so that we all can become more fully human, more enlightened, more liberated.

Nursing Education as Liberal Education Is Growth

Finally, and perhaps at its greatest, nursing education as liberal education is synonymous with growth. Dr. Dewey, as one of the 19th and 20th centuries' most influential philosophers and educational reformers, you contend that the goal of education is growth (Noddings, 2007, p. 26).

This stance confused others and they asked you, "Growth toward what?" Perhaps they too viewed education as an institution whose outcome was a precise way of life, similar to the psychologist and brick mason in DuBois's declaration. You adamantly insist that growth is its own end. Asking "growth toward what?" is incompatible with the conceptualization of growth. Specifying its path or target would make growth stiff and rigid. Growth leads to more growth.

I understand growth as a goal, Dr. Dewey. Growth, and hence education, is bigger than "producing a nurse." Growth seems similar to learning as the spirit that sustains me. That is, I never ask myself, "Learn what? What am I to learn?" Growth and learning are like my clematis vine in spring. Each delicate new stem wisps and curls as it wills, without shame, grasping the trellis that I devotedly burrow at its base every year. The clematis doesn't wonder, "Grow where? Grow toward what?" As the summer sun lures it up, the stretching clematis simply grows with a mind of its own.

But how do we satisfy the current emphasis on outcomes in education? Our legislators, as well as educational administrators, parents, students, and the public—even our professions—demand an outline of educational outcomes. Most of us have weathered (or is it "withered"?) through hours of meetings and pages of wordsmithing to fill, once again, the tabula rasa of education objectives. And yet, Dr. Dewey, you tell us that the goal of education is growth, plain and simple?

Perhaps, in an effort to appease, we need to do both, for now at least. First, we must list the specific aims of education inherent in preparing a person as we teach life, and second, we must realize that preparing a person, at its finest, is awakening and uplifting that growth. Of course, we know that the process of listing particular educational outcomes—filling the tabula rasa—can be invaluable in awakening our own growth as we dialogue with others.

Awakening our own and students' growth requires both *time* and *action*. Time is needed for discovery. Students need time to explore and play and fumble as amateurs without our hasty assessment of their spontaneity or our premature critical appraisal of their work in progress.

I continue to mull over what constitutes time for students' learning and what time is necessary for our evaluation of students. For example, too often we hurriedly evaluate students as they practice clinically, without providing ample time for their learning and their blundering. We expect them to be nurse experts while they are learning. We rush to closure and overlook the quintessence of staying power, of patience. To be honest, my husband and I have taken ballroom dance lessons for several years and yet we are still neophytes because we botch the same swing steps time and time again. Likewise, in both clinical and classroom teaching, the discovery process demands time and time again.

In awakening our students' growth, action and movement also call for attention. For instance, moving tables and chairs in the classroom encourages students to move about the room. A student once protested, "I can't stand classes where we all sit in rows and stare at the teacher. It makes me feel like a trained seal." In the same way, then, it must be safe for everyone to move among different ideas, to change in the process of discovery.

How can we help students talk with each other, rather than "train" student–teacher dialogue? How can we help students discover ideas, move among ideas, connect ideas? In choosing a single phrase depicting the essence of a liberal education, William Cronon (1999) picked E. M. Forster's ruling: "Only connect." Nursing education as liberal education finds the unexpected, sees quirky patterns, and unearths odd connections. Undeniably, we cannot connect if we are trained as seals, we cannot connect unless we have time, unless we act and move.

In his recent book *The Assault on Reason*, Al Gore (2007) expands the notion of movement and relates it to a plea for a collaborative conversation among all citizens. He argues that today most of the information flow is in one direction. "The world of television makes it virtually impossible for individuals to take part in what passes for a national conversation. *Individuals* receive, but they cannot send. They absorb, but they cannot share. They hear, but they do not speak. They see constant motion, but they do not move themselves" (p. 16).

If we value growth as the goal in liberal education, we must create safe space for time and movement. This safe space for teaching and learning needs to be spared, at least to some extent, from the vulnerability of day-to-day life. When I'm having a really good day as an educator, I'm able to take and sift thought and word, keeping what is precious and blowing the rest away with a breath of kindness—even if it is with just one student. I am still learning what it is that is worth keeping and what can be gently blown away. And that learning is the spirit that sustains me. For me, Dr. Dewey, that learning is growth.

IN PROCESSION: WHERE IS IT LEADING US?

In *Three Guineas*, Virginia Woolf (1938) responds in a series of letters to three requests, each from a different society asking her for money. One of the societies was a women's college building fund, which was a metaphor for family college funds that sent boys but not girls in the family to college.

In responding to this request, Woolf bemoans the sagging and mechanical education of the times and its lifeless results and, of course, laments the gender inequality. In her description of this education and its consequences, she imagines a procession: a "procession of the sons of educated men . . . educated at public schools & universities, mounting those steps, passing in and out of those doors, ascending those pulpits, preaching, teaching, administering justice, practising medicine, transacting business, making money . . . most of them kept in step, walked according to rule" (pp. 60–61). In Woolf's account, one can hear the programmed, mindless clacking cadence of the individual students and graduates, as well as the education system itself.

Today, as in the time of Woolf's writing, comparable processions march forward in our nursing education and healthcare systems. Some of them are gorged with compliance and conformity, exacting cheerfulness and enthusiasm. In other processions, nurses who have been prepared "to work" keep in step, pass in and out of those same doors, and walk according to those same rules. Diluted educational cobbling shadows still other processions, where students and faculty count courses and keep score—and little more. In all of these, the processions crimp the students and brutally sculpt them to fit in an inward-looking healthcare system.

As a start, we must ask ourselves, Are we trudging and rambling in any of these processions? Do we even see behind what we are traipsing? Woolf (1938) admonishes us, "Do we wish to join that procession or don't we? On what terms shall we join that procession? Above all, where is it leading us?" (p. 62).

In reshaping nursing education as liberal education, existing processions plead for our scrutiny—a courageous and comprehensive examination by new and emerging faculty. Knowing the self, relating vigilantly with students, and designing deliberate teaching practices contribute to that scrutiny. Art, agency, and growth will further guide us to study the procession, choose our membership, and determine where it is leading us.

In this scrutiny, we must stop taking our cues from old legends. Instead, we must proclaim a new story as our legacy, a new song as our anthem, a new path for our procession.

REFERENCES

Bevis, E. O., & Watson, J. (2000). *Toward a caring curriculum: A new pedagogy for nursing.* Sudbury, MA: Jones and Bartlett.

Cronon, W. (1999). "Only connect": The goals of a liberal education. *Liberal Education, 85*(1), 6–12.

DuBois, W. E. B. (1986). *Writings.* New York: Literary Classics of the United States.

Ehrenreich, B. (2001). *Nickel and dimed: On (not) getting by in America.* New York: Henry Holt and Company.

Ehrenreich, B. (2005). *Bait and switch: The (futile) pursuit of the American dream.* New York: Henry Holt and Company.

Gore, A. (2007). *The assault on reason.* New York: Penguin Press.

Greene, M. (2001). *Variations on a blue guitar: The Lincoln Center Institute lectures on aesthetic education.* New York: Teachers College Press.

Hersh, R. H., & Merrow, J. (Eds.). (2005). *Declining by degrees: Higher education at risk.* New York: Palgrave Macmillan.

Hitchens, C. (2001). *Letters to a young contrarian.* New York: Basic Books.

Noddings, N. (2007). *Philosophy of education* (2nd ed.). Boulder, CO: Westview Press.

Otsuka, J. (2002). *When the emperor was divine.* New York: Anchor Books.

Pausch, R., & Zaslow, J. (2008). *The last lecture.* New York: Hyperion Books.

Randy Pausch will now take your questions. (2008, April 21). *Time, 171*(16), 4.

Shulman, L. S. (2004). *The wisdom of practice: Essays on teaching, learning, and learning to teach.* San Francisco: Jossey-Bass.

Tolan, S. (2006). *The lemon tree: An Arab, a Jew, and the heart of the Middle East.* New York: Bloomsbury.

Trimble, J. R. (1975). *Writing with style: Conversations on the art of writing.* Englewood Cliffs, NJ: Prentice Hall.

Whyte, D. (1994). *The heart aroused: Poetry and the preservation of the soul in corporate America.* New York: Doubleday.

Woolf, V. (1938). *Three guineas.* San Diego, CA: Harcourt Brace Jovanovich Publishers.

The Musicality of Teaching: More Dreams for the Future Than Memories of the Past

Not perfection as a final goal, but the ever-enduring process of perfecting, maturing, refining is the aim of living.

—John Dewey

When I introduced this book I proposed grace notes as a metaphor for its foundation. Grace notes, as the ornaments of music, decorate the principal notes and augment the beauty and vigor of the work. As a grace note, I hope that my discussion has built on your clinical proficiency and distinctive personhood to help you embrace nursing education and affirm you as a new nurse educator. Further, I hope that I've been able to *show* you something, maybe even begin to show you the touchy and tricky spots *sideways*, on the *slant*. I hope that I did not stress *telling* you things or telling you things bossily.

Here I'm called to have my final say, to synthesize, to gift the reader as you return to everyday teaching. From that angle, I could say once again, "Please remember to pause and examine who you are as a person and a nurse educator and to connect with students, with learning, and with nursing education as liberal education."

THE MUSICALITY OF TEACHING

Instead I wish to return to music as an ending watermark. John Dewey's ever-enduring process of perfecting, maturing, refining as an educator stirs us to develop the "musicality" of teaching. This musicality of teaching is the ability to *hear* and the nerve to *convey* one's self and the discipline of nursing. The musicality of teaching is listening, understanding, pulling, and at the same time, it is speaking, revealing, pushing. It is not the precise note or rhythm, the strict technique or the how-to. Rather, the musicality of teaching teases out the tone of who we are . . . and that is the teaching ultimate.

155

I hear the *musicality of teaching* when a student writes in her e-mail message, "You were the first person I thought of, you have always thrown me a lifeline." But I know that I missed when I'm not able to hear the students' perspective about a flawed test item or a duplicate assignment or classroom strategy that just didn't fly. I also hear the *musicality of teaching* when alumni tell me about the research-mindedness they create in their work settings. But the musicality flattens when I've lost the courage to advocate for a minority voice, even though I believe that voice is sound. I hear the musicality of teaching when, after class or clinical or an interaction with an individual student, I am able to smile on the inside as well as on the outside. All of these tease out the tone of who I am and all of these are the ultimate of teaching.

Furthermore the *musicality of teaching demands a lifetime.* Teasing out the tone of who we are follows a forever twisting thread of fatigue, daily-ness, mistakes, repetition, and patience—a delicate and fragile thread, yet a crystal one just the same. This thread "bares" the ever endurance of John Dewey's edict.

Some may think this grasp on the brittle thread a foolhardy devotion, but it is like a change of season, a flower blossoming. As you look intently, staring, never taking your eyes away for one minute, there is no change. But glance away momentarily and look back again, and the leaves are open in Spring, colored in Autumn. The petals of the blossom glow, reds and yellows, as Summer slides out and Autumn slides in.

Still more, the *musicality of teaching demands a lifetime of looking forward.* In his recent book *The World Is Flat,* Thomas Friedman (2005) claims that perhaps the most important measure of a society, in addition to employment, life span, and literacy rate, is whether that society has more memories of the past than dreams for the future. These dreams for the future are the dreams of John Dewey: perfecting, maturing, and refining ourselves to tease out who we are as educators. Friedman quotes an organizational consultant who says, "One thing that tells me a company is in trouble is when they tell me how good they were in the past. Same with countries. You don't want to forget your identity. I am glad you were great in the fourteenth century, but that was then and this is now. When memories exceed dreams, the end is near" (p. 451).

Others also have championed the importance of looking forward. In guiding new writers about the limiting back-story in fiction writing, Stephen King (2000) advises, "As a reader, I'm a lot more interested in what's *going* to happen that what already *did.* . . . I like to start at square one, dead even with the writer. I'm an A-to-Z man; serve me the appetizer first and give me dessert if I eat my veggies" (p. 227). From another viewpoint, Moaveni (2005) exposes past memories some of the old Iranian aristocratic families held during the Revolution who withdrew into themselves and "tried to protect the cultivated grace of their lost world from being tainted. . . . Inside, time stood still" (p. 144).

Our world in nursing education is changing from once upon a time. Nevertheless, what hopeless memories of the past do we grip? Might these memories also be part of our lost world that cement us to stand still? And might we only be *imagining* that the world then was cultivated or graceful? What are we air-brushing out of the picture?

These memories may expect all nursing students to look, act, and dress alike or they may link all students with parallel personal, family, and cultural backgrounds. Might these memories drag all students down a harshly set educational track as one cohort with exact clinical and classroom experiences, allowing exceptions only with a celestial intercession? Yet, is there one way for a nurse to *be*? Do numbers of hours, or a precise pattern of clinical settings, or a specific sequence of classes signify a sought-after standard? To what extent do these clutched memories grind down a liberally educated individual?

Like the memories we may hold about students, I'm also learning that we expect (or even require) some nursing faculty to earn certain graduate degrees with a specific focus and conduct predetermined research. Further, we may be rewarding one way of teaching and learning. Perhaps in our effort to mature and refine, we believe in one identity cloned from one mold, copied from one pattern.

Those may be our memories. In our dreams for the future, as we refine our musicality, we cannot stammer in our notes or stutter in our techniques. We cannot allow our memories of the past to eclipse our dreams for the future.

BUILDING BRIDGES

In my dreams for the future, I see nurse educators scaffolding students to build more bridges. We must teach students to build bridges between technology and design, between the details and the big picture, between the function and the aesthetic, between causes and effects.

For example, we must teach students to build bridges between health care and planet sustainability. In the past, the focus has been health care; more recently, sustainability is the focus. We must dream the bridge between them. That is, how might we help others see and live the connection between a vegetarian diet, health care, and planet protection? Additionally, what is the relationship between health, the mammoth meat consumption in the United States, and the deaths from hunger caused by global warming and drought in Darfur or the Democratic Republic of the Congo?

In addition, we must teach students to build bridges between technology, effectiveness, and efficiency. I recently trudged with a family member through our healthcare system, with a modest insurance policy in one hand and an educated and capable problem-solving skill set in the other hand. Yet the gaps in our system emerged as enormous.

I have a small example—trivial, perhaps, but with ballooning consequences. Within a few short months, all within the same local healthcare system, I was asked at least two dozen times to give the family member's history of allergies, medications, surgical and medical interventions, and current signs and symptoms. I wanted to melt in fury by the seventh or eighth time I was asked for written replies to the same questions or responses to an assistant's queries about these exact items. Time and time and time again, I reasoned, "As technology escalates, the clock ticks, and healthcare dollars mount, why are all these precious resources shrunken with all of this duplication?" What I needed most of all was help with managing eldercare in our home to prevent high-priced institutionalization. Although I was given a handful of brochures and assorted pamphlets from the Office on Aging, extended with a sympathetic look and a kindly comment, I was left empty-handed and exhausted. But yet I was asked, once again, about allergies and cause of father's death, and year of last tetanus shot.

We must educate students not to only provide care, but to change care. I dream for the time when our students merge technology, effectiveness, and efficiency so that they can indeed provide care because they have changed the system, and patients and families receive what they need.

In another dream-bridge, we must educate students to move beyond "thinking globally and acting locally." We must *act* globally, not merely *think* globally. Global action relates to global poverty, politics, education, and health care, and it may or may not begin with a local awareness. Global action must be immediate and deliberate. I am convinced we cannot wait for local action first.

This conviction surfaced from a Native American student as I tried to "preach" the simple to complex idea to her, an idea that I did not question at the time, and neither did most of my colleagues or established curricular circles. I thank Kim for her brazen and bold contention: "I need to see the big picture first, the holism. Please don't begin by just telling me about a leaf or a prairie flower, a caterpillar or a pinecone. I need to first honor the earth and sky, the day and the night all as one." My dream, then, is for all of us to act globally. I must first see and teach students to see the earth and sky, the day and the night as one.

As we educate students to build these bridges we will need both the day and the night to refine our musicality of teaching. I'd like to borrow from Dr. Lee Shulman's (2004) use of Shakespeare to wish you "calm seas and auspicious gales" as you tease out the tone of who you are. As you spot the dreams you have for yourself and the students, for teaching and global health, may you have the security of still waters, tranquil reflection, and quiet composure. And may you also have the promise of changing winds, the stirring of unforeseen storms, and the vibrancy of growth and learning.

A closing farewell: Late one blank and icy December night as I grappled with this book's conclusion, I anguished to my husband, Wayne, "What should I write?" With his usual candor, goodwill, and sparkling smile, he said, "Just say thanks for reading my book." So, with Wayne's flair and energy, I say to you, "Thanks for reading my book."

REFERENCES

Friedman, T. L. (2005). *The world is flat: A brief history of the twenty-first century.* New York: Farrar, Straus and Giroux.

King, S. (2000). *On writing: A memoir of the craft.* New York: Pocket Books.

Moaveni, A. (2005). *Lipstick jihad: A memoir of growing up Iranian in America and American in Iran.* New York: Perseus Books Group.

Shulman, L. S. (2004). *The wisdom of practice: Essays on teaching, learning, and learning to teach.* San Francisco: Jossey-Bass.

Index